DRUG RELATED PROBLEMS
IN GERIATRIC NURSING HOME PATIENTS
James W. Cooper, PhD, FCP, FASCP

SOME ADVANCE REVIEWS

This book is timely for health professionals with responsibilities for drug management in long-term care facilities and nursing homes. With years of experiences in patient drug management, the author reveals the improper as well as proper procedures relative to geriatric patient care. Specific types of drug-related problems are abundantly covered as are case studies which illustrate the author's many points. So too are the responsibilities reviewed for the attending physician, nurse, consultant pharmacist, nursing home administrator, and other health professionals for the management of drug and nutritional services for the elderly. For all who are concerned about proper pharmacotherapy for the older patient, regardless of place for care, this book is a must.

Heber W. Youngken, PhD
Dean Emeritus
College of Pharmacy, University of Rhode Island

This insightful book is filled with facts, anecdotes, observations, and case studies making it lively reading. Dr. Cooper's book gives practical suggestions on the application of pharmaceutical care to the elderly. This useful book provides pharmacy practitioners, educators, and students with useful insights, critical questions, practical suggestions, and valuable guides to provide pharmacy services to the elderly in general, not just to nursing home patients.

Fred M. Eckel, MSc
Professor and Chairman
Division of Pharmacy Practice, The University of North Carolina

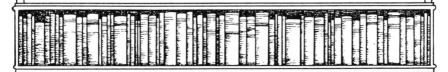

Drug-Related Problems in Geriatric Nursing Home Patients

PHARMACEUTICAL PRODUCTS PRESS
Pharmaceutical Sciences
Mickey C. Smith, PhD
Executive Editor

New, Recent, and Forthcoming Titles:

Principles of Pharmaceutical Marketing, 3rd Edition edited by Mickey C. Smith

Pharmacy Ethics edited by Mickey C. Smith, Steven Strauss, John Baldwin, and Kelly T. Alberts

Drug-Related Problems in Geriatric Nursing Home Patients by James W. Cooper

Pharmacy and the U.S. Health Care System edited by Jack E. Fincham and Albert I. Wertheimer

Pharmaceutical Marketing: Strategy and Cases by Mickey C. Smith

International Pharmaceutical Services: The Drug Industry and Pharmacy Practice in Twenty Major Countries of the World edited by Richard N. Spivey, Albert I. Wertheimer, and T. Donald Rucker

Drug-Related Problems in Geriatric Nursing Home Patients

James W. Cooper, PharmPhD, FASCP

Pharmaceutical Products Press
New York • London • Sydney

Pharmaceutical Products Press, 10 Alice Street, Binghamton, NY 13904-1580
EUROSPAN/Haworth, 3 Henrietta Street, London WC2E 8LU England
ASTAM/Haworth, 162-168 Parramatta Road, Stanmore (Sydney), N.S.W. 2048 Australia

Pharmaceutical Products Press is a subsidiary of The Haworth Press, Inc., 10 Alice Street, Binghamton, NY 13904-1580

Library of Congress Cataloging-in-Publication Data

Cooper, James, 1944-
    Drug-related problems in geriatric nursing home patients / James W. Cooper.
        p.   cm.
    Includes bibliographical references.
    Includes index.
    ISBN 1-56024-085-7 (alk. paper). — ISBN 1-56024-086-5 (pbk. : alk. paper)
    1. Geriatric pharmacology. 2. Nursing home patients. 3. Drugs — Side effects. I. Title.
[DNLM: 1. Drug Therapy — adverse effects. 2. Drug Therapy — in old age. 3. Nursing Homes. WT 100 C777d]
RC953.7.C66 1990
615'.704 — dc20
DNLM/DLC
for Library of Congress   90-15615
                                                                                            CIP

Dedication

This book is dedicated to all older persons who have used medications, sometimes with less than optimal results, specifically, the patients who have been harmed by the occurrence of drug-related problems that went undetected, went unresolved, or were ascribed to other causes. Personally, this book is dedicated to my maternal grandparents, Mary Alice Ray and William George Boston, and my paternal grandparents, Sarah Lou Newsom and Warner Rowe Cooper.

CONTENTS

ALL PHARMACEUTICAL PRODUCTS PRESS BOOKS
AND JOURNALS ARE PRINTED
ON CERTIFIED ACID-FREE PAPER

ABOUT THE AUTHOR

James Cooper, PharmPhD, FASCP, is Professor and Head of the Department of Pharmacy Practice at the University of Georgia College of Pharmacy in Athens, Georgia. He is the author of over 200 research and professional publications and the editor of the *Journal of Geriatric Drug Therapy* and *Clinical Consult*. He teaches, practices, and conducts research in consultant clinical pharmacy with geriatric patients in ambulatory and long-term care settings. Dr. Cooper is a fellow of the American Society of Consultant Pharmacists and was special advisor to the White House Conference on Aging.

Foreword

This book is intended to help pharmacists, physicians, nurses, and administrators who deal with nursing home patients, and health care planners realize the possible scope and magnitude of drug-related problems in nursing home care.

The results published in this book were first published in the inaugural issue of the *Journal of Geriatric Drug Therapy*[1] and expanded on, in part, in a series of articles which appeared in *Nursing Homes and Senior Citizen Care*. My clinical practice, research, and teaching results during 17 years in 9 nursing homes in the South and New England, the evolution of the disciplines of clinical and consultant pharmacy, and the always helpful comments of my colleagues and students have helped to make this book possible. I hope that not many nursing homes share the frequency of medication mishaps presented in this text and that those who consult on the appropriate utilization of drugs in long-term care may benefit from this text. The practical resources and methods developed for detection and resolution of drug-related problems (DRPs) are available in another text.[2] The specific results demonstrate the significance of the problems of drug usage in one nursing home.

The goals of this book are to make both health care planners and practitioners aware of the scope of DRPs, and patient/family rights and responsibilities, as well as to propose a higher standard of care for optimal medication usage in older adults.

Each chapter details methodology, references, and results, as well as practical detection, intervention, and resolution checklists. Illustrative cases also help the reader to put the results into a practical context.

Caveat: This book is not intended to replace sound medical judgment. It is intended to ensure that all medical judgments regarding medications are rational and understandable by all persons responsible for the patient.

James W. Cooper

REFERENCES

1. Cooper JW. Drug-related problems in geriatric long term care facility patients. *J Ger Drug Ther* 1986; 1(1):47-68.

2. Cooper JW. Community and Nursing Home Drug Monitoring Guidelines. Consultant Press, Watkinsville, GA, 1991.

Acknowledgement

The encouragement and support of my wife, Susan Eure, and the patience of my children, Jay and Allison, made this book possible. Unfortunately, the medication misadventures depicted in this book did occur, but hopefully they do not typify all long-term care pharmacotherapy of nursing home patients.

Chapter 1

Drug-Related Problems in the Elderly at All Levels of Care

SUMMARY. Drug-related problems (DRPs) are more common in elderly than in younger patients. Drug-related problems may contribute to up to one-third of hospital and one-half of nursing home admissions of elderly patients. Within institutional care settings, both medication errors and adverse drug reactions are a significant source of increased morbidity and mortality in older patients. Swing bed, home health, day care and ambulatory geriatric patients have frequent problems with their medications. Identification of the at-risk patient, further evaluation of the effect of multidisciplinary interventions in DRPs, and significant funding initiatives to find cost-effective methods to prevent and decrease the frequency of DRPs should be priority goals of gerontology and geriatrics education and research programs. Families and patients should be aware of the magnitude of these DRPs and be able to seek logical answers to determine when there is a drug-related problem, as well as the most rational ways to resolve and prevent the DRP.

INTRODUCTION

Drug therapy is the most frequently utilized treatment modality in the elderly. While other modalities of nutrition, psychosocial, and physical activities play vital roles in the total (holistic) care of the patient, the likelihood of a drug causing problems that worsen the prognosis of the patient is greater than with any other modality of treatment.

1

DEFINITIONS

Drug-related problems (DRPs) may be defined as any unwanted consequences of the drug utilization process. Although many events can and do occur in this process, from the assessment of a patient's problems to the therapeutic outcome in that patient, the two main DRP classifications are drug misuse and adverse drug reaction or interaction. When both types of problems are simultaneously assessed in the same patient population entering a hospital, the frequency of those problems has been demonstrated to increase with age.[1] The purpose of this chapter is to characterize the frequency of and factors associated with DRPs in the elderly at all levels of care.

ADMISSIONS TO HOSPITALS AND IN-HOSPITAL DRPs

When a complete history of drug use prior to admission is done on all patients entering hospitals by consulting with the patient's community pharmacist, one of every five admissions has been associated with a DRP, when all age groups are combined. Almost one-third of patients age 65 or older had DRPs that influenced their need for admission. Two-thirds of these problems were drug misuse, especially underuse of needed medications, and one-third of DRPs were adverse drug reactions and interactions to prescribed therapy taken as ordered.[1]

The most important factors (% of patients) associated with drug-related problems were:

1. Lack of patient knowledge of prescribed therapy (47.6) — The patients could not answer three simple questions regarding their medications: "What is/are the name(s) of your medications?" "What is each medication supposed to do for you?" and "How are you supposed to take your medications?"
2. Inability to afford the medication (32.3) — Patients had to choose between paying for their needed drugs and food, rent, or utilities.
3. Physician and pharmacist lack of knowledge that a DRP had influenced the patients admission (88).[1]

Once in the hospital, almost one-third of patients over age 65 had an adverse reaction, based on the medical services in over 10,000 patients studied in 9 hospitals around the world. This rate is slightly higher than that of the general hospital population.[2] A national sample of medication errors found that 12.2% and 11.0% of doses in nursing homes and hospitals, respectively, were given in error, with omission of needed doses and administration of unauthorized drugs accounting for most of those serious drug misuse errors.[3]

NURSING HOME ADMISSIONS AND LENGTH OF STAY PROBLEMS

An average of three DRPs per patient was found on 50 consecutive admissions to a nursing home. Paradoxically, only one-third of the patients' total medical care problems had been identified before admission to the facility. Medication misuse, unnecessary therapy, therapy needed for newly identified problems, adverse drug reactions, and missing lab and physical data needed to evaluate drug therapy were the most common DRPs.[4] The DRPs identified were considered the cause of admission in over one-half (26 of 50) of the cases. Once patients were in the long-term care facility, rigorous drug regimen reviews conducted monthly by regulatory mandate found significant DRPs of drug misuse and adverse reaction and interaction in 65% of the cases.[5]

The involuntary termination of these rigorous drug regimen review services has been associated with doubling of drugs per patient and an increase in DRPs and death rates. Subsequent reinitiation of these drug regimen services in the same facility has been found to lower admission, discharge, and death rates and to cut drugs per patient in half.[6] In all three studies, the factors associated with DRPs were failure to adequately document patient problems and follow rational pharmacotherapeutic principles, ignoring stated DRPs brought to the prescriber's attention, and lack of intensive diagnostic work-up and follow-up on the patients.[4,5,6]

The swing bed concept has been proposed as an alternative method of handling geriatric patient transition from the hospital to the nursing home. A recent study of swing bed patients found that within a 20-day average length of stay, 65% had an adverse drug reaction, and 60% of patients exceeded their per diem total care allowance in drug costs alone within the first 3 days of their swing bed admission.[7] The apparent reasons for the DRPs noted were, again, incomplete work-up, failure to adequately monitor patient progress, "dumping" patients prematurely when all of their Medicare hospital days had been used up, and mismatching patients with this level of care.

HOME HEALTH AND DAY CARE PROBLEMS

Home health patients have significant DRPs of misuse in over one-half of cases evaluated. The most common DRPs were stopping or changing doses without professional consultation when the patient was on needed chronic care medication.[8] Similar findings were noted in an older adult day care study.[9] At both levels of care, the apparent reasons for the problems were a lack of patient knowledge and comprehension of both disease states and pharmacotherapy, lack of thorough evaluation of patient status and therapeutic progress, and perceived lack of pharmacist and prescriber interest in the care of the patient.

AMBULATORY PATIENT PROBLEMS

In a recent study of drug-related problems in a multiple site ambulatory geriatric population, 53.4% of patients had significant DRPs. Misuse and adverse drug reaction were, again, the most common problems. Patient misperception of drug knowledge and prescriber and pharmacist lack of detection of drug-related problems by thorough drug regimen review were factors associated with these problems.[10]

The checklist in Figure 1-1 should serve to let each caregiver, patient, patient's family, or responsible party determine knowledge of the care of the patient. If any of the questions cannot be adequately answered, then it is the responsibility of the individual(s) to get those answers, write them down, and carry them to each health

Figure 1-1

Caregiver/Patient/Family Checklist for Conditions and Drugs

1. Do I know all disease states and conditions and understand what these diagnoses mean for my future?_____

2. Do I know all drugs ordered on both regular and as needed bases for my diagnoses?_____

3. Do I know how all my drugs are to be given and why they are given this way?_____

4. Do I know why each drug is ordered and for what diagnosis it is intended to treat?_____

5. What is each drug likely to do for me when I take it; or when I refuse to take it?_____

6. Does my physician make sure that I understand all my diagnoses and other medical problems?_____

7. Does my pharmacist make sure that I understand all my medications and keeps a record of all my drugs, both prescribed and purchased without a prescription, such as remedies or patent or over-the-counter medicines? _____

8. Do I keep an index card with all my diagnoses and drugs to show to my physician and pharmacist, and check with either before taking any other drug they have not prescribed or filled? _____

9. Am I aware of the drug-related problems that can or have affected me or my family member and the consequences of the DRP?_____

10. Do I have one primary care physician, who approves of any new therapy ordered by any consulting physician; do I have one primary care pharmacist, who ensures that my medications are safe to use together ?_____

11. Do any other caregivers, such as dentists, podiatrists, physical therapists, dieticians or social workers know my history?

care provider the patient sees. This should help to ensure that everyone knows what should occur in the care of the patient.

IMPLICATIONS AND RESEARCH QUESTIONS

It appears from this brief survey of existing drug-related problem studies that these problems are quite common in the elderly at all levels of care. This chapter does not purport to be a complete review of the area, but it does emphasize papers that used similar methodologies, operational definitions, and classifications. There are a number of valid research questions and recommendations to be raised from this review:

1. Why are drug-related problems so prevalent at all levels of care? Should larger-scale studies be done, using similar rigorous methods to identify, quantify, and find methods to reduce this prevalence?
2. What are the educational, socioeconomic, psychological, and quality of medical care ramifications of drug-related problems?
3. What interventions are most cost-effective in identification and reduction of drug-related problems?
4. What funding initiatives should be encouraged from private and public groups that should be responsive to these issues?
5. How can health care practitioners work together to identify and reduce drug-related problems in their respective practices?
6. How can elderly health care consumers become more aware of the magnitude of drug-related problems and more active in their own preventive self-care?
7. What can patients do to improve the quality of their self-care?

REFERENCES

1. Frisk PA, Cooper JW, Campbell NA. Community-hospital pharmacist detection of drug-related problems upon patient admission to small hospitals. *Am J Hosp Pharm* 1977; 34:738-742.

2. Miller RR. Drug surveillance utilizing epidemiologic methods—a report from the Boston Collaborative Drug Surveillance Program. *Am J Hosp Pharm* 1973; 30:584-592.

3. Barker KN, Mikeal RL, Pearson RE, et al. Medication errors in nursing homes and small hospitals. *Am J Hosp Pharm* 1982; 39:987-991.

4. Cooper JW. Effects of intensive consultant pharmacy review of nursing home admission orders. *Consult Pharm* 1987; 2:152-155.

5. Cooper JW. Drug-related problems in geriatric nursing home patients. *J Ger Drug Ther* 1986; 1(1): 47-68.

6. Cooper JW. Effect of initiation, termination, and re-initiation of consultant clinical pharmacist services in a geriatric long-term care facility. *Med Care* 1985; 23:84-88.

7. Cooper JW. Drug-related problems in swing-bed patients. *Consult Pharm* 1988; 3:257.

8. Cooper JW, Griffin DL, Francisco GE, et al. Home-health care: drug-related problems detected by consultant pharmacist participation. *Hosp Form* 1985; 20:643-650.

9. Cooper JW. Drug-related problems in day-care patients *Consult Pharm* 1988; 3:193.

10. Wade WE, Cobb HH, Cooper JW. Drug-related problems in a multiple site ambulatory geriatric population. *J Ger Drug Ther* 1986; 1(2):67-79.

Chapter 2

Drug-Related Problems
in the Long-Term Care Facility

SUMMARY. The purpose of this chapter is to overview the types of drug-related problems that can occur in a long-term care facility (LTCF). Drug-related problems (DRPs) are defined as any unwanted or unintended consequences of the administration or nonadministration of medications. There are two general types of DRPs: (1) misuse by any person associated with drug prescribing, filling, administration, and assessment and (2) adverse drug reactions and interactions.

A recent two-year study[1] of DRPs in LTCFs found that up to two-thirds of drug regimen reviews (DRRs) revealed a significant DRP in this patient population. Subsequent chapters in this book deal with the DRPs found in this population and significant factors associated with misuse. Figures 2-1 and 2-2 detail the problem list and drug regimen review process used in this study. An explanation of individual acronyms and symbols can be found in the legend. Figure 2-3 gives examples of significant DRR findings with bogus names but actual problems found in a subgroup of patients on one monthly review. Each patient's suspected DRPs were identified to the attending physician through the Director of Nursing of the facility. The right column is used for physician and/or nurse follow-up to problem identification by the consultant pharmacist. Completed copies of each monthly and quarterly summary of consultant pharmacist reports were retained in a binder for state Medicaid licensure and medical care foundation on annual inspection of the facility.

Figure 2-1 Clinical Pharmacy Service Patient Problems List

Patient Name-Jane Doe _____ Doctor-Smith_____

Age/Ht.Wt/Race/Sex-73yo5'4"145lb.WF___ Adm. Date-8/87_____

Adm.PE-ROS-VS__BP 170/98_____ Adm.ABN Labs-K=3.3_____

Date Prob.No. Active Problem*   TX/Rx Plans/Results Date to S/P

9/87   1. HBP Maxzide-25 i daily B/P 128/72_____

3/88   2. Osteoarthritis ECASA 10grs QID No c/o pain_____

5/88   3. Glaucoma Betoptic 2gtts OU BID   IOP <20_____

6/88   4. Constipation MOM 30 ml QON   No impactions_____

7/88   5. Depression Norpramin 25mg QAM Better socializaiton

(etc.,etc. for as many problems are noted......)

*Problems include established diagnosis, physiological/physical

change, symptom/sign, lab test or physical abnormality, psycho-

logical or socioeconomic problem, med error, past oper-

ations/procedures, adverse drug reactions/interactions and

compliance with therapy. S/P signifies status-post, or past event

that should be kept.

Figure 2-2 Drug Regimen Review Procedure/Checklist

    1. Obtain and establish data base from chart

    2. Write a problem list and match therapy with problems

    3. Evaluate therapeutic goal attainment by checking for:

    a. Medication errors

    b. Drug interaction or adverse reaction

    c. Compliance by nurse, patient, doctor, pharmacist,
       family and facility

    d. Need for education/inservice for any in c.

    e. Data sufficiency for drug efficacy and toxicity evalua-
       tion

    f. Optimal/economical drug therapy being utilized

    4. Complete drug regimen review and document and communicate
       pertinent findings.

Figure 2-3 Some Examples of Drug Regimen Review Findings

Patients of Dr. Jones   at : Local Nursing Home

Patient Name	Findings/Recommendations	Response/Results
Jane Doe	Not receiving over 1/2 of doses for high blood pressure and heart failure, with elevated BP and increased edema noted.	Inservice and Incident reports for charge nurses- one dismissed.
Sam Smith	Patient received ferrous sulfate and antacid together, and anemia still unimproved.	Schedule antacids 2 hrs. after meals and Hgb/Hct increase documented.
Dina Diabetic	Patient and family not adhering to diabetic diet. Blood sugars >300 mg/dL noted with 13 pound weight gain past 3 months.	Patient/family re-education and warning that patient will be dismissed if not compliant.
Tin Blood	Patient on Coumadin with no Pro times, appears anemic and black stools noted	Pro time ordered bi-weekly and Coumadin dose decreased.
Low Globin	Patient appears anemic, but not on iron and taking NSAI	Stop NSAI, start hematinic

A summary of DRPs found over the two-year period can be found in Table 2-1. Specific operational definitions and drugs involved each category are detailed in Appendix A. This study has detected a far higher incidence and period prevalence of DRPs than earlier studies. There is no accepted model for DRR in long-term care facilities. The indicators for assessment of DRR in LTCFs are, at best, very minimal standards. This introductory chapter is by no means an attempt to establish optimal standards. This is merely an attempt to document in an anecdotal fashion the results of intensive DRR in one LTCF. The questions of immediate importance to con-

Table 2-1

Drug-Related Problems Detected in a 72-Bed Nursing Home Over 24 Months

Categories	No. (%) of Problems	Example
1. Medication Administration and Documentation Errors	324 (26.5%)	Omission of Regular Scheduled Antihypertensives blood pressure increased 20-30/10-20 mm Hg.
2. Relative Contraindication.	202 (16.5%)	Use of KCl in patients with moderate renal impairments (CrCl < 50 ml/min) and serum K greater than 5 mEq/L.
3. Adverse Drug Reaction or Interaction	161 (13.1%)	Suspected digoxin toxicity with anorexia, digoxin held due to pulse < 60 and digoxin level > 2 ng/ml. Antacids given with iron salt or tetracyline, anemia still present or bronchitis not improved.
4. Nutritional/Hematinic Consideration	128 (10.5%)	Patient with consistent weight loss not on restricted caloric intake or who had serum albumin < 3.5 Gm/dL or total lymphocyte count < 1500 especially if decubitus or chronic UTI/catheter present.
5. Socioeconomic Consideration	124 (10.1%)	Patient/Family unable to pay for medication-recommendation of less expensive alternative therapy.

Categories	No. (%) of Problems	Example
6. Drug Duplication	78 (6.4%)	Multiple antipsychotic use in patient with dementia.
7. Questionable Drug Efficacy	47 (3.8%)	Papaverine use in dementia.
8. Therapeutic Need by History but Treatment Modality not ordered	46 (3.8%)	History of glaucoma.
9. Lab test or Blood level need to assess Drug Therapeutic/Toxic end point	42 (3.4%)	Request serum potassium in patient with Hx hypokalemia on furosemide and digoxin. Digoxin level request in suspected toxicity.
10. Dosing Interval/Schedule Simplification	24 (2.0%)	Drug with > 24 hour half-life dosed qid.
11. No established diagnosis but drug used or used inappropriately.	21 (1.7%)	Antidepressant prn for sleep or depression.
12. Patient Refusal/Inability to take chronic care medication	18 (1.5%)	Refusal to take antihypertensive with blood pressure increase.
13. Dosing Modification/ length of therapy or change to drug with shorter half-life	9 (0.7%)	Request use of shorter rather than longer half-life benzodiazepine in patient with abuse history and carryover sedation.

————————

1224 (100%)

sultant pharmacists, nursing directors, medical directors, and administrators in the LTCF are:

1. How well are DRPs detected in my facility?
2. How are DRPs documented, assessed, and followed up on by persons capable of problem resolution?
3. How do the types and frequency of DRPs found in this study compare with our facility?
4. How does DRP detection, documentation, assessment and resolution follow-up lead to improved patient care?

Figure 2-4 is a checklist for general adequacy of DRR in a LTCF. Subsequent chapters will have similar checklists for each type of DRP.

```
Figure 2-4 Drug Regimen Review Adequacy Checklist

        Does the consultant pharmacist :                    Yes   No

Review the entire patient chart on LTCF admission?          ___  ___

Write an initial problem list on each patient to be

retained in chart and/or then patient records?             ___  ___

Match the problem list with all therapies ordered

to determine rationale, need and coverage of problems?     ___  ___

Observe how the patient responds to each drug in terms

physical(vital signs) and lab (e.g. serum electrolytes,

hemaglobin/hematocrit) findings?                           ___  ___

Check for medication errors and verify drug administration

and documentation by comparison of dispensing records

with the medication administration records (MAR)?          ___  ___

Make written notation of suspected DRPs in a monthly

report to nurses and physicians involved in patient care?___  ___

Does the Director of Nursing:                               Yes   No

See that all attending physicians get a copy of recommenda-

tions?                                                      ___  ___

Coordinate follow-up response to problem detection and resolu-

tion?                                                       ___  ___
```

Ensure that charge nurses are involved in
DRP detection and resolution? ___ ___

    Does the attending physician: Yes   No
Acknowledge the consultant pharmacists communication when a written copy of consultant pharmacists
report is sent to their office? ___ ___
Respond to consultant pharmacist or director of nursing communications regarding drug therapy? ___ ___
Make any changes in patient therapy in response to consultant
pharmacist or nursing communication? ___ ___
Encourage consultant pharmacist input to the evaluation
of the patient? ___ ___

    Does the Patient and Their Family or Responsible Party:
Understand their rights to know their disease states and conditions? ___ ___
Understand the need for each medication being used in the
patient, and any risks and benefits of each drug? ___ ___
Understand what lab and physical assessment is being done to
monitor their disease states/conditions and therapy? ___ ___
Understand that the nurse, physician and pharmacist are
responsible for making sure that the patient is properly treated
and followed and can explain anything not understood to the
patient and/or their responsible party? ___ ___

REFERENCE

1. Cooper JW. Drug-related problems in a geriatric long term care facility patients. *J Ger Drug Ther* 1986; 1:47-68.

APPENDIX A

Drug-Related Problems Operational Definitions

A. Medication administration and documentation errors — The presence of a difference between doses dispensed and those documented given; omission; wrong drug, dose, or schedule; or documentation error that could affect the intended therapeutic goal attainment, with evidence of detrimental or less than optimal patient treatment response (e.g., omission of regularly scheduled antibiotic with resultant worsening of acute bronchitis in patient with chronic obstructive pulmonary disease).

B. Relative contraindication to drug use — A patient with a history or established diagnosis that would necessitate the reevaluation of the use of the current drug therapy, due to the potential for an adverse reaction (e.g., order to digitalize patient in congestive heart failure who had pulse 32-36 BPM and ECG evidence of 3° heart block).

C. Nutritional/hematinic need assessment — Defined as the patient with:

1. Consistent undesirable weight loss with or without prior caloric restriction (e.g., diabetic)
2. Inability to eat, poor appetite, or unwillingness to eat
3. Chronic infection (e.g., chronic urinary tract infection)
4. Anemia, (Hgb < 12 Gm/dL in either sex) or trauma, decubitus ulcer, or fracture; or with the
5. Laboratory value of serum albumin < 3.5 Gm/dL, total lymphocyte count < 1500 and/or hemoglobin/hematocrit < 12/36
6. Insufficient caloric amount or protein intake with multiple vitamin and appropriate minerals (e.g., iron for iron deficiency or blood loss anemia other than anemia of chronic disease or senescence, zinc for wound healing, calcium for osteoporis-related fractures) to ensure positive nitrogen balance and weight maintenance or gain as appropriate
7. The patient who was above these lab values whose weight had attained or exceeded prior usual or ideal weight, decubitus ulcer or fracture was healed, or chronic infection was not present
8. The patient who did not show therapeutic response of improvement in weight, healing, or lab parameters despite nutritional therapy and was considered to need reevaluation of nutritional/ hematinic therapy.

D. Socioeconomic consideration — Defined as the patient/family who was unable to pay for needed medication, and, therefore, less expensive alternatives (e.g., specific drug that was on Medicaid formulary, generic equivalent, or a combination product that incorporated two or more single agents) were available.

E. Adverse drug reaction or interaction—Defined as presence of an unwanted response to a single drug that necessitated the discontinuance of that drug (e.g., ampicillin itching rash), a decrease in the dose (e.g., tranquilizer oversedation) an alteration in the dose schedule (e.g., flurazepam no more often than every third night due to carryover daytime sedation or use shorter acting benzodiazepine), or addition of another drug (e.g., KCl in diuretic-associated hypokalemic hypochloremic metabolic alkalosis). A drug-drug interaction was defined as the concurrent use of two or more drugs that may produce an adverse reaction, actual or predictable, or alter the desirable therapeutic response (e.g., concurrent digoxin and furosemide with a serum K/Cl 3.5/95 mEq/L and patient complaints of nausea, palpitations, and "funny colors in my eyes").[a,b,c]

F. Drug duplication—Use of more than one drug with the same pharmacological properties for a problem usually treated with a single agent in variable dosage (e.g., multiple antianxiety and/or antipsychotic drugs for patient with dementia).

G. Questionable drug efficacy—Defined as drugs classified "less than effective" or "probably ineffective" by the National Academy of Sciences/Drug Review Council[a] or by established clinical practice[b] (e.g., papaverine in dementia or methenamine in acute urinary tract infection (UTI) or chronic UTI with urine pH > 6).

H. Therapeutic need by history but no treatment ordered—Defined as the patient with a history of an active problem or established diagnosis with no treatment ordered for the problem and patient signs, symptoms, or lab test indicating continued need for therapy (e.g., patient with history of glaucoma with complaints of chronic headache and steadily diminishing vision with no treatment ordered for glaucoma).[c]

I. Lab test or blood level needed to assess drug therapeutic/toxic end point—Defined as the need for laboratory test or drug serum level when any combination of signs, symptoms, patient disease, drug, drug dose, or prior lab work indicated prudent need for objective evaluation.

J. No established diagnosis but drug used or used inappropriately for established diagnosis—Defined as the absence of documentation of established diagnosis (e.g., dementia), use of drug for signs or symptoms (e.g., restlessness or agitation), or not allowing appropriate time period for therapeutic evaluation (e.g., doxepin prn depression).

K. Patient refusal or inability to take chronic care medication—Defined as an omission shown to be detrimental to the patient. Prescriber awareness is essential for reevaluation of the patient before subsequent treatment orders are given (e.g., patient with angina pectoris-associated chest pains who refuses sublingual, oral, or topical nitroglycerin due to severe headaches).

L. Dosing interval or schedule change that would improve patient compliance, therapeutic response, and/or administration rate, or diminish side effects—Defined as multiple daily dose administration where drug half-life is greater than 24 hours (e.g., antipsychotics), simplification of multiple daily dose schedule (e.g., 4 to 2 times or once per day) where therapeutically acceptable (e.g., methyldopa), giving antimicrobials (except sulfonamides and nitrofurans) a.c. and drugs with gastric irritant potential pc., and changing time of day drug is administered to minimize side effects (e.g., thioridazine h.s. only where daytime sedation is a problem).

M. Length of drug therapy or half-life consideration—Defined as (1) exceeding the manufacturer's recommended length of therapy (e.g., cimetidine full dose QID greater than 6 to 8 weeks) or (2) drugs with long half-lives are used daily for longer than recommended (e.g., daily diazepam, propoxyphene, and/or flurazepam in patients with history of abuse or worsening dementia when agent is started).

a. *USPDI* Vol. 1, Easton, PA: Mack Printing Co., 1984.

b. Katcher, BS, Young, LY, Koda-Kimble, MA, eds. Applied therapeutics. 3rd ed. San Francisco: Applied Therapeutics, Inc..

c. Mangini, KJ, ed. Drug interaction facts. St. Louis: J.P. Lippincott, 1985.

Chapter 3

Communication of Drug-Related Problems Within the Nursing Home

SUMMARY. Effective communications between the consultant pharmacist and patients, patients' families, and the attending physician, as well as nursing home personnel, are reviewed. Communication components of clinical significance/severity, coordination, continuity, and culpability are detailed, and case examples of types of communication recommendations are given.

COMPONENTS OF CLINICAL COMMUNICATIONS

There are at least four components to communications in the nursing home: clinical significance/severity, coordination, continuity, and culpability. Clinical significance of patient findings can be put into a hierarchy of increasing significance: potential, possible, probable, and documented. For example, a patient with an order for Valium® prn agitation gets daytime sedation and has trouble sleeping. The evening charge nurse calls the attending physician, who orders Dalmane® to be given prn sleep difficulty. The consultant pharmacist recognizes a *potential* for an adverse reaction from the two benzodiazepine drugs that should probably never be used in the elderly due to their long half-lives of residence in the body (7 to 20 days).

SIGNIFICANCE HIERARCHY

The consultant pharmacist or charge nurse may call the attending physician or write a recommendation to discontinue (d/c) both drugs before more serious problems of excessive sedation occur. If

19

the attending physician is not aware of the situation with two long-acting anxiolytics, the patient may develop oversedation as a *possible* consequence of the use of both relatively contraindicated drugs. When either drug is used daily, alone or in combination, there is a high likelihood of a *probable* adverse reaction.

The *documented* adverse reaction is where the offending agent is discontinued, and the patient gets better (dechallenge), or another long-acting anxiolytic (Paxipam®, Tranxene®, Librium®) is substituted, and the identical oversedation problem develops with daily use (rechallenge). If, in fact, some degree of chemical restraint is needed for the patient's, other patients', or facility's protection, a shorter-acting agent (Serax®, Ativan®, Restoril®, Xanax®, Halcion®) is preferred, unless psychotic symptoms of dementia mandate a relatively nonsedating antipsychotic (Haldol®) in low doses (less than 2 mg per day).

SEVERITY HIERARCHY

The severity of drug-related problems should always be recognized when a drug-related problem is suspected in the nursing home patient. Most adverse reactions to drugs are mild in that they are bothersome side effects of the medication, not usually necessitating a significant change in the drug regimen. For example, the sedation caused by most antihistamines (e.g., Benadryl®) is bothersome and can be anticipated by discontinuance of other sedating drugs while the antihistamine is being used for allergy, colds, hayfever, or sinus problems.

Most nonsteroidal anti-inflammatories (NSAI) (e.g., Feldene®, Motrin®, Naprosyn®, Clinoril®, Tolectin®, Orudis®, Meclomen®, Voltaren®, Ansaid®, Dolobid®, Arthropan®, Disalcid®, Moban®, Trilisate®, and aspirin) used for arthritic pain can cause stomach distress to acute stomach bleeding if not taken with food or a dose of antacid. A drug-related problem of moderate severity involves the need for some change in drug therapy. The patient who regularly takes a NSAI is very likely to develop anemia as a consequence of prolonged NSAI treatment (3 to 6 months or longer). The detection of falling hemoglobin/hematocrit levels (Hgb/Hct), which should be done every 2 to 3 months in the patient on chronic NSAI therapy, signals the need for discontinuance of such therapy or a switch to an analgesic (e.g., acetaminophen, enteric-coated aspirin) that is not associated with the development of anemia. The best alternative if the patient truly has an inflammatory (reddened, hot, or swollen joint) arthritic pain (rare in the elderly LTCF patient) is the use of enteric-coated aspirin, which rarely causes anemia.

At least 95% of the drug-related problems detected by the consultant pharmacist or evaluated on the suggestion of the charge nurse/ director of nursing in the LTCF are of minor to moderate severity. Major severity denotes a life-threatening event involving the toxic effects of medication in the patient. If no action was taken when patient complained of GI upset when the NSAI was given, the patient goes on to develop probable NSAI-associated anemia (which could also have been detected by regular Hgb/Hct determinations, inspection of the conjunctiva, and checking stool color) and is admitted to the hospital with massive GI bleeding, more than likely associated with the NSAI. Recognition of this problem early in the minor stage could avoid a life-threatening event. How often does the consultant pharmacist or nurse detect or suspect a problem that goes unheeded until the probability of a major adverse reaction is apparent?

LEGAL AND RESPONSIBLE PARTY CONSIDERATIONS

It should be apparent to the family or responsible party of anyone placed in the nursing home when a change has occurred in the alertness, mentation, or general well-being of the patient. Once a question is raised regarding this suspected change, the charge nurse is responsible for making an entry in the "nursing notes" of the question raised, with whom the nurse discussed the problem, and the resolution of the problem to the satisfaction of the person raising the question.

Since the patient's chart is a legal document, the responsible party or the party's attorney should have access to the chart, with or without a court order, to assure the adequacy of the care of the loved one. Most nursing home administrators will assure families of their right to know and understand the basis for any action taken in the care of the patient.

PREVENTIVE CARE

It is abundantly clear that nursing homes have to be centers for preventive care as well as for after-care in cases of acute problems. To establish the rehabilitative aspect of care, the LTCF administrator must be assured that the consultant pharmacist services not merely meet, but exceed the minimal indicators that are the federal standard. No administrator wants to run a facility that is known as a dying or a dumping place for patients. There is no patient who wants to be in such a facility nor is there a family that wants its loved one to be in such a place.

DIAGNOSIS-RELATED GROUPS (DRGs), DUMPING, AND SWING BEDS

The advent of diagnosis-related groups (DRGs) for acute care reimbursement on a fixed cost basis means that LTCFs must be prepared for sicker patients who need a markedly greater level of care, especially in the areas of nutrition, medications, and physical therapy. Many health care practitioners have witnessed the premature "dumping" of the patient from the hospital, where the DRG reimbursement limits or Medicare days have been exceeded, to the nursing home with limited care capability and subsequent poor outcome.

Swing beds, in the hospital with a less than 100% census, have been proposed to serve as a transition from the acute to the long-term care facility. A recent study of drug-related problems in geriatric swing bed patients demonstrated that perhaps "dumping" is still a problem, especially where there are inadequate reimbursement mechanisms for the swing bed care.[1]

COMMUNICATION COORDINATION

Coordination of clinical communications in the LTCF is perhaps the most difficult component to effectively administer, yet it is the vital link among the individual physicians, charge nurses/aides, nursing supervisor and director, consultant and vendor pharmacists, medical director, and administrator. Tragically, the most significant and severe problems may go unnoticed and unattended, and dire consequences may result when no one assures coordination of communication.

An actual case from a consultant pharmacist's experience illustrates extreme lack of communication coordination. The consultant pharmacist noted an 88-year-old black female with high blood pressure who on monthly drug regimen review had: Dyazide® one BID; KCl 10% 15cc in juice daily and a low-sodium diet; pulse 46-60; BP 90/54-114/68; and complained to the nurse of extreme weakness, lethargy, and inability to carry out the activities of daily living for the past month. It was 11 PM at night when the review of medications was done, and the consultant pharmacist tried to call the attending physician without success. The on-call covering physician refused to do anything about the situation and told the consultant to call the physician the next day during office hours. On completion of his review, the consultant left a written report with the director of nursing (who was on leave) and a note for the charge nurse to call the physician's office the next morning to request a serum potassium. The consultant would be on business in the next town and unable to call from that location. The note to the charge nurse was lost, and the nursing director was out of town on leave for a week. On recheck, the consultant found that no action had been taken and called the physician's office and had to leave a message because the physician was not in. The massage came to the attention of the physician by the end of the day, but the KCl was left off, and the doctor stopped the Maxzide® but not the KCl. The patient became progressively stuporous and obtunded with pulse 32 to 40 BPM. The physician finally ordered a serum potassium two weeks late, which turned out to be 7.2 mEq/l (normal range 3.5-5.0 mEq/l). The physician ordered Lasix® and Kayexalate® but did not stop the KCl until the consultant finally reached him personally and asked him why the KCl was needed if he was using the Kayexalate® to lower serum potassium.

It may appear at times that "Murphy's Law" rules situations that occur in the LTCF. On discussion of this case with the attending physician, the physician frankly revealed that he received a lot of insignificant and nonurgent calls after hours that prompted his office staff to believe that most calls from this particular LTCF were not that important.

The LTCF administrator must be assured, along with the director of nursing and the consultant, that there is a definite communication coordination protocol that is followed and followed up on with some degree of continuity.

COMMUNICATION CONTINUITY

Continuity of clinical communications refers to everyone knowing how the protocol for communications works and continually follows that protocol. Each facility should have a defined protocol for when to call the attending physician, depending on the urgency of the problem. A constipated patient or one who has difficulty sleeping is not usually cause for a call outside office hours, but if this type of event occurs, just as in the preceding example, there is not likely to be sufficient attention to significant patient care problems. Some facilities, for instance, specify that the charge nurse may not directly call the doctor unless a distinct emergency or life-threatening event is occurring with the patient.

Continuity usually requires that the nursing supervisor or director of nursing review and evaluate the problem before a call is made. While there are many ways of handling nonemergency drug-related problems, some may prefer routine orders for pain, constipation, temperature, diarrhea, coughs and colds, and lab work as needed. Although federal and state regulation forbids this, many facilities have de facto routine orders as a result of a number of standing and/ or prn orders for drugs and lab work. There is a balance between good medical practice and writing an order for every possible event that could occur in the patient.

When the consultant pharmacist makes observations and gives his monthly or quarterly report, the LTCF administrator should be assured that the components of clinical significance/severity (and urgency), coordination, and continuity are apparent, because every consultant recommendation must be communicated to the individual attending physicians, and some notation of receipt by the doctor must be given to the facility for its records. Medicaid regulations do not require the doctor to make any changes or to take any action in response to these recommendations, but the doctor must at least acknowledge receipt of these recommendations.

Should there be a lack of response or failure to take any responsible action on the part of the attending physician, the Medical Director may have to be consulted for arbitration and judgment on significant problems to protect the patient. The final component of communications deals with culpability or responsibility for patient care.

CULPABILITY OR "WHERE THE BUCK STOPS"

Culpability rests upon the administrator, medical director, director of nursing, and consultant pharmacist for seeing to the doctor taking care of patient drug problems and other care-related problems. In this litigious society, with families admitting their loved ones to nursing homes with a tad of guilt in many cases, there is fruitful ground for many a lawsuit for errors of omission or commission by the facility. Attorneys have been known to subpoena both the chart and consultant pharmacist recommendations to determine if they have grounds for a suit against the facility. Both state and federal inspectors want to see, in many inspections, both consultant recommendations and evidence of follow-up by the physician and facility.

Examples of consultant pharmacist recommendations and physician acceptance of those recommendations is indicated in Table 3-1. The two-thirds acceptance rate gives some indication of the significance of the problems and the willingness of the individual attending physicians to accept these unsolicited, but needed, consults on their patients. Subsequent chapters will detail specific types of drug-related communications and problems and give case-management techniques used in individual situations. A checklist is found in Figure 3-1.

Table 3-1

Consultant Recommendation Acceptance Rate (%) (Action taken)

		Nurses	Physicians
1.	Medication Errors	324/324 (100%)(Incident Report)	
2.	Relative Contraindication to Drug Use	150/202(74.3) --	(D/C drug and/or change to non-contraindi-cated drug in same drug group
3.	Adverse Drug Reaction and Interactions (ADR andI)	20/20(100)	113/141(80.1) (D/C or change drug schedule,dose, or order drug to treat ADR)
4.	Nutritional/Hematinic Assessment	--	93/128(72.7) See operational defini-tions in app.A,Ch.2
5.	Socioeconomic Consideration	---	43/124(34.7)(D/C (D/C Drug or use com-bination product)
6.	Drug Duplication	---	51/78 (65.4)(D/C Drug)
7.	Questionable Drug Efficacy		42/47 (89.4)(D/C Drug)
8.	Therapeutic Need	---	40/46 (87.0)(Order Drug)
9.	Lab Test/Blood Level Needed	---	40/42 (95.2)(order test or level)
10.	Dosing Interval Change	---	10/24 (41.7)(Order drug to be given fewer times/24h)
11.	No Established Diagnosis or inappropriate use of drug	---	5/21(23.8) (D/C drug)
12.	Patient Refusal/Inability to take drug	---	5/18 (27.8)(Change dosage form or drug or D/C drug)
13.	Dosing Modification	---	4/9 (33.3)(Change to recommended drug)

	Nurses	Physicians
Sub-total	344/344 (100%)	596/880 (67.6)
Total	930/1224 (76%)	

Figure 3-1

<u>Patient/Responsible Party Communications Checklist</u>

1. Does the charge nurse always let me know when a problem exists ?____

2. Does the physician let me know when there is a problem and its resolution ?_____

3. Is the consultant pharmacist available to explain any communication problem regarding drug therapy ?_____

4. Does the nursing home have a good reputation for communication follow-up, continuity and culpability ?_____

REFERENCES

1. Cooper JW. Drug-related problems in a geriatric long term care facility. *J Ger Drug Ther*, 1986; 1:47-68.

2. Cooper JW. Drug-related problems in geriatric swing bed patients. *Cons Pharm*, 1988; 3:83.

Chapter 4

Drug-Related Problems in Nursing Homes: Medication Errors

SUMMARY. Medication errors committed by nursing home personnel include omission, wrong dose, wrong drug, wrong schedule, extra doses, documentation error, and improper stop-order procedures. They are the most frequent DRPs encountered in the nursing home. The purpose of this chapter is to discuss the implications of a study of medication errors in one LTCF over a two-year period. The most common types of medication errors, case reports, and cost analysis of specific medication errors will be presented. A checklist for preventing medication errors for all health care practitioners and patients and their families is essential to identifying and reducing the prevalence of this DRP.

A comprehensive study of drug-related problems (DRPs) in one nursing home recently found that two-thirds of drug regimen reviews (DRRs) detected a significant DRP.[1] The most common DRP in over one-fourth of the cases was a medication administration or documentation error. Table 4-1 details the type of medication errors, drug classes involved, and rank order of occurrence of both error and drug class.[1]

The methods used to detect medication errors, in this study were:

1. Monthly review of each patient's medication administration record (MAR) for doses signed off, correct transcription of medication directions, and drug administration times as part of the monthly DRR;
2. A comparison of the doses dispensed and signed into the facility with refill dates for the past 30 days;

3. Observations of the medication nurse for one medication pass during the medication pass that occurred while the monthly DRR for the facility was conducted; and
4. A thorough review of the treatment book for sign-off and notation of patient response to the treatment.

Table 4-1*

Medication Errors in One Nursing Home Over a Two-Year Period

Type	total(%)	Nutr	GI	GU	Antiinf	CV	Endo	Topical	NSAI	Neuro
				Drug Classes Involved						
Omission	211(65)	56	28	5	8	62	15	29	4	4
Extra Doses	28(8.6)	3	6	-	10	7	2	-	-	-
Wrong Dose	20(6.2)	-	12	-	-	3	1	-	2	2
Wrong Drug	6(1.9)	2	2	-	2	-	-	-	-	-
Unordered Drug	10(3.1)	1	2	-	-	5	-	1	1	-
Doses Not Signed Off	49(15)	4	6	-	4	5	2	22	2	4
Totals	324	66	56	5(	24	82	20	52	9	10
(%)	(100)	(20.4)	(17.3)	(1.5)	(7.4)	(25.3)	(6.2)	(16.1)	(2.8)	(3.0)

*Note: An error was assigned for each patient case where monthly review found that DRP.

Nutr=nutritional or hematinic supplements(e.g.FeSO4)

GI=gastrointestinal drugs (e.g. cimetidine)

GU=genitourinary drugs (e.g. propantheline)

antiinf=antiinfectives(e.g. ampicillin)

CV=cardiovascular meds(e.g.propranolol)

Endo=endocrine drugs(e.g.insulin)

topical=dermal treatments

NSAI=non-steroidal antiinflammatory drugs(e.g. ibuprofen)

Neuro=neuroactive drugs (e.g. thioridazine)

As may be noted in Table 4-1, almost two-thirds of the medication errors were omission, followed by doses not signed off (but presumably given), extra doses, wrong doses, unordered drug, and wrong drug. The specific drugs involved; the apparent reasons for each type of error; and the consequences for the patient, the nurses, and the facility deserve further presentation and discussion to help the nursing home administrator, director of nursing, and consultant pharmacist to anticipate, detect, and prevent such errors in their facilities. Patients and their families or responsible parties need to be aware of common medication errors, their prevention, and their resolution.

OMISSION ERRORS

Failure to give a dose of medication as ordered is by far the most common type of medication error in both acute and long-term care facilities. The best way to prevent such errors or any type of DRP in the LTCF is some type of unit-dose or modified unit-dose system for the patient. Unit-dose is a prepackaged supply of drug in 24-hour to 30-day supply with retention of drug identity (usually as unit-dose packaging) until the drug is administered to the patient. All doses of medication are also accounted for in a true unit-dose system, whether it is 24-72 hour, or modified weekly to monthly refill system. If the period of use is greater than 72 hours, some prefer to refer to this system as a "modified" unit-dose system. The essential element, whether 24-hour or otherwise, is unit-of-use accountability (i.e., each dose is accounted for).

The pharmacist who supervises the filling and refilling of individual drug orders is the ideal person to assure that drugs are given as ordered, when this professional regularly communicates with the nurses administering the drugs to the patients of the nursing home. Such communication, which was the subject of the last chapter, may help to determine what problems are evident and, with the cooperation of the attending physician and administrator, can help to resolve these drug administration problems.

In a recent study, the patients of one facility were served by seven different pharmacies and had an eighth pharmacist who was the consultant pharmacist and did not have an association with any of the seven pharmacies. In addition, there was not a unit-dose system of any kind in use. Drug refills were called into the individual pharmacies rather than refilled via an automatic cart exchange process. Drug quantity for each drug filled and refilled was verified by the charge nurse on duty for that floor or wing. This tedious process, which is necessary when a unit-dose system is not in use, can consume as much as 8 to 12 nursing hours per 100 beds per week in the LTCF and is subject to a much higher rate of medication errors.

The drug classes involved in omission may again be noted in Table 4-1. Specific cases or generalized examples illustrate the significance and severity of the omission of these drugs. Multiple vitamins and iron salts were the most frequently omitted medications. The apparent reasons for the omissions were patient refusal due to drug-associated gastrointestinal (GI) upset, ranging from nausea with vitamins to constipation with iron salts.

In most cases, the charge nurse, rather than marking "refused" on the MAR, simply failed to give the drug. To handle this problem it is essential that both drugs be given with food to minimize GI upset. Unfortunately, the reason for giving the vitamin was poor food intake, so unless the patient is given sufficient water or antacid with vitamins the patient's nutritional state is not improved. Antacids cannot be given with iron salts, as the antacid ties up the iron and prevents its absorption. GI products such as antacids were not refilled often enough to be given correctly. Tagamet® bedtime doses were omitted due to the patient sleeping at the hour; unfortunately, the patient's stomach ulcer, which the Tagamet® is supposed to prevent from recurrence, flared up, and the patient had to be transferred to the hospital for acute gastrointestinal bleeding. The cost of this medication error was $8,500 for the unnecessary hospitalization.

Anti-infective omissions were perhaps the most serious. A 78-year-old black male patient with chronic lung disease had amoxicillin 250 mg tid prescribed, and half the doses were not given over a 7-day period for his acute bronchitis. The patient was hospitalized for 4 days, was given the same drug via the same route over this time, and was readmitted to the LTCF, with a hospital bill for $3,923. Omitted cardiovascular medications included digoxin, antihypertensives, and antianginals, with four further needless hospitalizations as a result.

A case of serious omission of medications serves to illustrate this problem. An 88-year-old white female with high blood pressure (HBP) received only two-thirds of her antihypertensives for the prior month and suffered from elevated BPs of 168/98 to 192/110 mm Hg. and had 4 transient ischemic attacks (which she had not previously developed). The apparent reason for this omission was that the patient was sleeping when afternoon to evening medications were to be given, and the charge nurse made the decision that the patient's sleep was more important than the HBP medications. Endocrine medications omitted were antidiabetics in oral dosage forms.

Significant omission of topical medications primarily concerned decubitus ulcer treatments in the afternoons, when the 3-11 PM treatment nurse made the decision that the dressings did not need to be changed. Neurotropic drug omissions were, for the most part, with the bedtime use of antidepressants and the charge nurse not understanding that the drug had to be given in order to be effective for depression. There was a misperception that since the drug was given at bedtime that it must be a "sleeping pill."

The use of incident reports for the nurses involved in these omissions, with reasons for the error and sign-off by the director of nursing, medical director, and consultant pharmacist, may help to prevent these errors. Some states allow only a certain number of medication errors and require serious errors to be reported to the state board of nursing, which can suspend or revoke the nurse's license.

Unfortunately, the latest state and federal inspection guidelines do not even call for the surveyor to check for omission errors by comparing doses replaced/refilled to the facility by the provider pharmacist. The remaining types of errors to be discussed, which in this study constitute only a third or less of all medication errors, are only the proverbial "tip of the iceberg" of medication errors. The revision of the surveyor standards should logically incorporate checking the consultant pharmacist's drug regimen review reports for reconciliation of doses dispensed/signed into the facility with the MAR dose sign-offs.

DOCUMENTATION ERRORS

Failure to sign an MAR or treatment book is the most readily accessible evidence of poor patient care to the surveyor. If a dose or treatment is not signed off, it is assumed that it was not given by most surveyors. For purposes of this study, however, a distinction was made between doses not signed off and those not given. If these first two types of errors are considered one and the same, they account for over 80% of medication errors reported in this facility. The primary area of persistent failure to sign for one's work was in the topical treatment of decubitus ulcer patients.

It is extremely worthwhile for administrators, directors of nursing, and consultant pharmacists to note the type of patient who may fail to get medications as ordered: the patient with Alzheimer's disease, chronic/organic brain syndrome, or simply labeled demented (all used synonymously in this study). In other words, the patient who was least likely to report or verify suspected omission of dose or sign-off was the most likely to have such an error in care occur.

EXTRA DOSES OR DOSES GIVEN PAST STOP ORDER DATE

The third most frequent medication error was in noting a change in the number of times a day that a drug should be given (e.g., dosing schedule changed from three to two times a day) or in giving drugs, especially antibiotics, beyond their stop order date (i.e., because doses were not given as ordered during the stop order period). While generally a lesser problem than omission errors, these types of errors may also point to omission when extra doses past the stop order period are either given or signed-off and not actually given. In either case, there is a breakdown in the established procedure, combined with a lack of mental alertness by the charge nurse.

WRONG DOSES OF MEDICATIONS

Wrong doses occurred mainly with antacids, Dilantin® and Mellaril® suspensions, and Lanoxin® and Lasix® elixirs. The use of dosing cups rather than dosing syringes was the chief reason for the inaccurate dosing of these liquids, except for Mellaril®, Lanoxin®, and Lasix®. In these three cases, there was a visual error in determining the proper dose. Proper attention to liquid refills and providing the nurses administering the medication with dosing syringes, especially where the dose is less than 10 ml., are essential to the prevention of this type of medication error. A 67-year-old white male with dementia was given 100 mg 3 times a day rather than the 10 mg of Mellaril® suspension ordered. After one week on this excessive dose, the patient was semicomatose, developed four decubitus ulcers, and died from sepsis within one month of the one week of excessive sedative usage.

UNORDERED DRUG GIVEN TO THE PATIENT

The main reason for this type of error appeared to be either an error in transcription of the order (i.e., order was actually for another patient), or the nurse incorrectly giving the patient a drug for which there was not an order (e.g., Lasix®, Darvocet®, Tagamet®). Nursing discretion with *pro re nata* (prn) orders does not extend to drugs for which there is no order. In one patient, the unauthorized use of Darvocet® led to acute confusion which resulted in an unnecessary Mellaril® order.

WRONG DRUG GIVEN TO THE PATIENT

Four of the six cases of this error involved giving the wrong hematinic, vitamin, or antacid. The remaining two cases, however, were potentially very serious, as the wrong antibiotic was ordered. A Vibramycin® order (a tetracycline) was taken verbally or understood to be Vee-Cillin® (a penicillin) and the patient was allergic to penicillins and had a moderately severe penicillin allergic reaction requiring three days of hospitalization at a cost of over $5,000. The second wrong antibiotic was a pharmacist error in providing the wrong drug. Only by all persons responsible for medication prescribing, filling, dispensing, and administration giving their fullest cooperation can medication errors be prevented.

Checklists for the nursing home administrator, director of nursing, consultant pharmacist, and families and patients to detect and prevent medication errors are found in Figure 4-1.

Figure 4-1-Medication Error Checklist

1. Nursing Home Administrator-do/does our-

   a. facility have an up to date policy and procedure manual for drug use control ?

   b. director or nursing and consultant coordinate effective drug use control ?

   c. incident reports get follow-up for medication errors?

   d. facility have a modified unit-dose accountability system?

2. Director of Nursing--do we get-

   a. good drug use system support from pharmacy?

   b. charge nurses following established medication administration policy and procedure?

   c. excellent dose and sign-off accountability?

   d. incident reports as a basis for nurse retention, raise and termination proceedings?

3. Consultant Pharmacist--do we have--

   a. the most efficient and accountable system for drug-use control?

   b. nursing cooperation in following established policy and procedure?

   c. providers of medication who are other than the consultant ?

   d. if c. is the case, do the providers comply with policy and procedure?

4. Patient/Responsible Party--do I see--

   a. excellent cooperation in the provision and administration of medication ?

   b. usual refills of all meds on or about their expected date(s)?

   c. obvious med errors that are brought to the administrator and nursing directors attention with unreliable follow-up?

   d. an active ombudsman program of patient advocacy in the facility?

CONCLUSIONS

The purpose of this chapter was to review the recent finding of medication errors as the most common type of drug-related problem in the LTCF.[1] No administrator, director of nursing, or pharmacist wants to have an inspection that detects a significant medication error problem and face the possibility of a "condition" being placed on continued certification of the facility, much less face loss of certification due to medication errors. The only way to prevent this possibility is to have constant vigilance for the reliable administration of drugs within the facility. The use of firm administrative procedures to include incident reports, in-services, warnings, firings, and written documentation of the use of these procedures is mandatory. There are many patients' families who will use any mechanism possible (e.g., medication errors) to purge their conscience and/or the facility of any person whom they believe is not providing optimal care to their loved ones. The ombudsman program can be an effective adjudicator of problems where there appears to be an impasse between the responsible party and the facility. Figure 4-1 is a medication error checklist.

REFERENCE

1. Cooper JW. Drug-related problems in a geriatric long term care facility. *J Ger Drug Ther* 1986; 1:47-68.

Chapter 5

Contraindications to Drug Usage

SUMMARY. Contraindications to drug usage are the second most common drug-related problem (DRP) found in a recent two-year nursing home study. Antiarthritic drugs, potassium chloride supplements, potassium-sparing diuretics, anti-infectives, antacids, reserpine, long-acting benzodiazepines, barbiturates, thiazide diuretics, and digoxin were the drugs most commonly found to be relatively to absolutely contraindicated in this population. Methods to anticipate and prevent the use of contraindicated drugs include a complete history, a problem list, and sophisticated consultant pharmacist services in the nursing home.[1] A checklist of possible contraindications is important to the patient and the patient's responsible party, as well as to all persons responsible for the nursing home care of the patient (Figure 5-1).

TERMS

Contraindication is defined as the presence of some condition or history in the patient that indicates that a drug should probably not be used. There are two types of contraindications: relative and absolute. The relative contraindication exists when a drug may be needed, and there may not be readily available alternatives to that drug (i.e., the benefit of use outweighs the risk of toxicity). Another instance where relative contraindication exists is where the risk of toxicity can be minimized by careful monitoring to anticipate toxicity. For example, referring to Tables 5-1 and 5-2, NSAIDs are the most common relatively contraindicated drug in the presence of a history of peptic ulcer disease and/or past gastrointestinal (GI) bleeding. By careful monitoring of the hemoglobin/hematocrit of the patient using NSAIDs and by watching for nonspecific GI complaints, one may prevent the development of toxicity.

Absolute contraindication exists when under no circumstances should the drug be used because not only is it very likely that if the

Table 5-1

Some Relative to Absolute Contraindications to Drug Usage

Organ System/Problem	Drugs Implicated	Solution
Cardiovascular/ raise BP and worsen heart pain	Decongestants in high Blood Pressure (HBP) or angina pectoris or heart attack history	Avoid Usage of oral or topical agents-watch in combination with antihistamines
Cause fluid retention	NSAIDs in HBP or congestive heart failure (CHF)	Watch for water weight gain
Worsens heart block	Digitalis in chronic CHF with heart block	diuretics are more rational and less toxic
Pulmonary/ nervous,can't sleep	Theophylline or Trental in patient with caffeine diet	Decaffeineate diet
Gastrointestinal/ cause anemia and ulcers	Aspirin or NSAIDs in history of peptic ulcer disease or GI bleeding (also watch oral cortico- steroids)	Use acetaminophen or enteric coated ASA or watch for anemia if must use NSAIDs
Worsen reflux e.g. of stomach contents	Donnatal, Robinul in hiatal hernia or reflux esophagitis	Use antacids, Gaviscon
Impaction	Bulk laxatives in the incontinent patient who is not able to drink fluids	Use 70% sorbitol or milk of magnesia
Irritant Laxatives Dulcolax, Modane, Ex-Lax	Use in those with laxative toxic colon/colon cancer	avoid- use 70% sorbitol/MOM
Accumulate in renal failure	MOM or magnesium-containing antacids	Avoid--use 70% sorbitol

Organ System/Problem	Drugs Implicated	Solution
Can get into lungs and cause lipid pneumonia	Mineral oil, Haley's MO and Vick's or Mentholatum inhaled or insufflated into nose	"
Diabetes/increase blood sugar	Diuretics	Watch Potassium Status
	Oral prednisones make patient more brittle	Follow fasting blood sugar(FBS)
"		
Make low blood sugar harder to detect (mask symptoms) and prevent body defense	Beta blockers (Inderal, Lopressor, Corgard, Tenormin, Visken, Blocadren,Normadyne/Trandate)	Avoid if possible-use calcium blockers instead of beta "
Neuropsychiatric/ Cause or worsen depression or dementia	Beta Blockers and Sympatho-lytic antihypertensives,e.g. Aldomet, Wytensin, Catapres, Ismelin, Hylorel	Avoid if possible-use ACE inhibitors or calcium blockers instead
"	Darvocet/Wygesic, Talwin, Percodan/Percocet	Avoid-use oral codeine, morphine or methadone if terminal pain present
"	Sedating Antipsychotics such as Mellaril,Serentil, Thorazine	Use lowest dose possible, or use less-sedating Haldol or Prolixin
"		

Long-acting benzodiazepines Avoid-use shorter acting such as Xanax,
       Librium, Valium   Serax,Ativan and Halcion
   Paxipam, Centrax

                    (NOTE: this group preferably only
      also associated with greater frequency of falls and hip
  fractures, decubitus, with any sedative increases problems)

TABLE 5-1 (continued)

Organ System/Problem	Drugs Implicated	Solution
Renal/impaired function[2]	Aminoglycoside antibiotics, e.g. Garamycin.Nebcin,Amikin, Netromycin,Sisomycin	Avoid if possible-dose on the basis of lean body weight and renal function.
greater drug toxicity	Macrodantin. tetracycline, sulfas,Pyridium, Cipro,	lower dose or prolong dosing interval or avoid if CrCl too low

drug is used in a patient the outcome may be serious toxicity but there are more suitable alternatives to the drug. An example is the case of the patient who has third-degree heart block, congestive heart failure, and a low pulse rate, where the attending physician is attempting to digitalize the patient.

The purpose of noting contraindicated drugs is to bring about the most efficacious drug treatment with the lowest risk of toxicity. The cases noted in Table 5-2 which will be discussed are attempts to *prevent* DRPs from progressing to adverse drug reactions (ADRs). (The next chapter in this book deals with ADRs and how they are handled.) In other words, by detecting drugs that are relatively to absolutely contraindicated before they become adverse drug reactions, the administrator, director of nursing, medical director, consultant pharmacist, and attending physicians can improve the care of the nursing home patient.

METHODS TO DETECT DRUG CONTRAINDICATIONS

The simplest ways to detect drug contraindications are team (doctor-nurse-pharmacist) thorough review of the patient's history, especially drug use history, writing a problem list of both present and past diagnoses, and using a sophisticated drug-regimen review process. It may, however, be true that some facilities are called "nursing homes" because the nurses render most of the care that is given to the patients due to the abrogation of responsibility by the physician and lack of a sophisticated drug regimen review by the consultant pharmacist.

In other cases, the physician may ignore important communica-

Table 5-2

Relative to Absolute Contraindications to Drug Usage Found in 2-Year

Nursing Home Study [1]

Drug Class	Number (%)	Preexisting Condition/ Diagnosis
Nonsteroidal Antiinflammatory Drugs (NSAID)	62(30.7)	History of peptic ulcer disease with bleeding associated with NSAIDs
Potassium Chloride Supplements or Potassium Sparing Diuretics	48(23.8)	History of moderate to severe* renal impairment
Tetracycline, Nalidixic acid, Nitrofurantoin or Methenamine Complexes	41(20.3)	History of moderate to severe* renal impairment
Magnesium Containing Antacids or Milk of Magnesia	29(14.4)	History of moderate to severe* renal impairment
Reserpine, Longacting Benzodiazepines, or Barbiturates	15(7.3)	History/evidence of depression
Thiazide Diuretic	4(2.0)	Creatinine clearance less than 10 ml/min
Digoxin	3(1.5)	Second to third degree heart block, pulse less than 50

202(100.0)

*Per W.M. Bennett, et al. Drug Prescribing in Renal Failure: Dosing Guidelines for Adults. Am.J. Kid. Dis., 1983: 5:155-193.
Reprints: The National Kidney Foundation, 2 Park Ave., New York, NY 10016, ($3.00)

tions in cases relative to absolute contraindications to drug usage. Again, as stated in Chapter 3, it is imperative that the administrator and director of nursing, along with the medical director, be assured that clinically significant DRPs brought to the attending physicians are acted upon to protect both the patient and the facility.

The alert patient or the responsible party may also be the person to point out relative to absolute contraindications to drug usage. Some illustrative examples of contraindications are noted in Table 5-2. This is not intended to be an all-inclusive list. The prescriber, pharmacist, nurse, and patient/responsible party should consult standard prescription product reference material (e.g., *Physicians Desk Reference*, also known as the *PDR*) or official compendia standards such as the *United States Pharmacopoeia Dispensing Information (USPDI)* for complete information.

A warning about the use of encyclopedic references such as the *PDR* or *USPDI* is in order. Many patients have a high degree of psychological suggestibility for symptoms or possible problems mentioned in these references. Too much knowledge about medications can deter compliant use of needed drugs for the heart, high blood pressure, diabetes, depression, ulcers, and other diagnoses that may require chronic drug usage for optimal drug benefit to the patient.

SPECIFIC CONTRAINDICATIONS CASES AND PREVENTION METHODS

The contraindications noted in a recent two-year study are listed in Table 5-2. The most common problem noted was the use of NSAIDs in the patient with a history of peptic ulcer disease (PUD), GI bleeding, or suspected history of the development of anemia while taking NSAIDs. The most common way that this contraindication is seen can be illustrated with a typical case (one of 62 noted).

An 84-year-old white female, 5'2", 277 pounds, with a history of osteoarthritis, PUD, anemia, and GI bleeding-associated hospital admission complains of joint pain to her doctor, who prescribes Naprosyn® 375 mg BID. After consulting the patient's problem list and noting that the patient had previously experienced anemia and GI bleeds with two other NSAIDs, the consultant pharmacist called the attending physician with this information. A change in the orders to cancel the Naprosyn® and start acetaminophen 650 mg PO QID was made, and the patient was counseled on the realistic expectations for pain relief that this drug could offer, as well as the consequences of prior NSAID use and the probable outcome (GI bleeding) if she could not tolerate the pain and insisted on her NSAID.

The second most common contraindication was the use of KCl supplements or potassium-sparing diuretics in the patient with history of moderate to severe renal impairment. This assessment was usually made on the basis of lab tests of serum creatinine (normal 0.5-1.5 mg/dl) which, if elevated, indicated the presence of renal impairment. Once creatinine in the serum increases over 1.5 mg/dl, there is a high likelihood that the kidney will retain more potassium, unless very potent loop diuretics (e.g., Lasix® or Bumex®) are being used to promote excretion of excess water and electrolytes. This is a relative contraindication, as the serum potassium should be kept between 4 and 5 mEq/l, and by frequent monitoring, one can see if an appropriate amount of potassium is being replaced.

The KCl supplements most commonly used are liquid KCl and the solid dosage forms Slow-K®, Micro-K®, K-Tab®, Klotrix® and Kaon Cl® tablets. The potassium-retaining diuretics are usually found in combination with the potassium-wasting diuretics as the combination products Dyazide®, Maxzide®, Moduretic®, and Aldactazide®. Appropriate cautions should also be exercised with the use of salt substitutes (e.g., Co-Salt®, Neo-curtasal®) in these patients. These condiments should never be used in the nursing home patient without an order and regular monitoring of serum electrolytes and renal function.

A case illustrates this point. A 73-year-old black male with a history of analgesic abuse and consequent analgesic nephropathy and kidney impairment had high blood pressure and serum creatinine on admission of 2.2 mg/dl. On screening the admission orders, which included Dyazide® one BID with no serum K, the consultant asked for serum electrolytes, which were sodium 128 (normal = 135-145 mEq/l) potassium 5.8 (normal = 4-5 mEq/l) and chloride of 98 (normal = 95-105 mEq/l) before the Dyazide® was restarted. On the basis of these findings, the physician changed the admission orders from low sodium to normal diet and from Dyazide® to La-six® 40 mg daily.

The third most common contraindication was the use of tetracy-cline, nalidixic acid (NegGram®), nitrofurantoin (Macrodantin®), or methenamine complexes (Mandelamine®, Hiprex®, Urex®) in patients with moderate to severe renal impairment. The use of a number of medications is relatively contraindicated when the body's ability to excrete these substances via the kidney is signifi-cantly decreased. A convenient way of classifying patient's renal function on the basis of their serum creatinine (ser cr) and their calculated creatinine clearance (CrCl) is as follows:

$$CrCl, ml/min (males) = 140 - Age/ser cr$$
$$CrCl, ml/min (females) = 140 - Age \times 0.85/ser cr$$

From this calculation a good approximation of both functional loss with age (140 - age) and organic loss of renal function can be made. For example, an 80-year-old female with a ser cr of 2.0 mg/dl would have a CrCl as follows: $CrCl = 140 - 80 \times 0.85/2 = 60 \times 0.85 = 30 \times 0.85 = 25.5$ ml/min. The calculated value will fall into one of the following ranges: (ml/min) Normal, $CrCl = 80\text{-}140$; Mild impairment, $CrCl = 50\text{-}80$; Moderate impairment, $CrCl = 10\text{-}50$; Severe impairment, $CrCl = $ less than 10 ml/min.

The patient example (25.5 ml/min) falls in the range of moderate renal impairment. There are other drugs that are relatively contrain-dicated in renal impairment, and either dosing adjustments or pro-longed dosing intervals must be used with these drugs, especially many antimicrobials, some antihypertensives, some NSAIDs, Diabinese®, Tagamet®, Atromid®, insulin, Benemid®, Anturane®, Mysoline®, allopurinol, and others (please see Bennett reference in Table 5-1).

The fourth most common relative contraindication was the use of magnesium-containing antacids or milk of magnesia in the presence of moderate to severe renal impairment. Maalox®, Gelusil®, My-lanta®, Riopan® all have magnesium which accumulates in ad-vanced kidney failure and can produce hypermagnesium-related symptoms of (if serum magnesium greater than 1-2 mEq/l) at 3-5 mEq/l hypotension, nausea, and vomiting; at 5-7 mEq/l, drowsiness, hyporeflexia, and muscle weakness; at 7-15 mEq/l, coma and heart block. The obvious way to prevent this problem from occurring is to watch for chronic renal failure (CRF) patients' use of standard antacids or MOM and switch them to non-magnesium containing antacids, such as Amphojel® or ALternaGEL®, and a different laxative, such as 70% sorbital solution.

Drugs associated with worsening or contributing to depression were the fifth most common contraindication. Reserpine in Hydropres®, Regroton®, Ser-Ap-Es®, Salutensin®, and Rauzide®; long-acting benzodiazepines such as Librium®, Valium®, Centrax®, Paxipam®, Dalmane®, Azene®/Tranxene®, and barbiturates such as Nembutal®, Seconal®, Tuinal®, Amytal®, and Butisol®; and phenobarbital and beta blockers such as Inderal®, Lopressor®, and Corgard® may all be associated with the problem. The use of antidepressants with any of these agents, especially when the antidepressant is started after the prior mentioned drug, suggests the possibility of drug-associated depression.

Thiazide diuretics generally do not work when the CrCl is below 30 ml/min., the sixth most common contraindication found in the study. Finally, digoxin should not be used in the patient with advanced bradycardia/heart block, due to the probable fatal consequences of such use.

Several other possible contraindications that may be common in many nursing home patients were not noted in this study. For example, the use of beta blockers in diabetic patients is relatively contraindicated due to masking of the effects of hypoglycemia and blocking of the release of sugar from the liver and muscle in low blood sugar conditions. Oral decongestants that do raise blood pressure are absolutely contraindicated in the high blood pressure patient but frequently go unnoticed when in combination with cold products such as with Ornade®, Drixoral®, Actifed®, Trinalin®, Dimetapp®, etc. For the concerned health care practitioner dealing with drugs, a simple procedure to check for contraindication would be to consult the *Physicians Desk Reference (PDR)* or product literature to ensure that a drug is safe to use with the conditions/diagnoses found in the nursing home patient. Figure 5-1 is a checklist for drug contraindication assessment.

Figure 5-1

A Checklist for Drug Contraindication Assessment

1. Does the facility have a complete drug history on each patient, to include past drug reactions ?

2. Does any patient have-

    a. impaired renal function

    b. impaired liver function

3. Is there as history of anemia, gastrointestinal bleed, sedation, depression or adverse drug reaction or interaction.

REFERENCES

1. Cooper JW. Drug-related problems in a geriatric long term care facility. *J Ger Drug Ther* 1986; 1:47-68.

2. Bennett WM, Singer I et al. Drug prescribing in renal failure: dosing guidelines for adults. *Am J Kid Dis* 1983; 3:155-193.

Chapter 6

Adverse Drug Reactions and Interactions in a Nursing Home

SUMMARY. Adverse drug reactions and interactions were the third most common DRPs in one nursing home. Neurotropic drugs followed by antihypertensives, potassium supplements, potassium-sparing diuretics, diuretics, digoxin, nonsteroidal anti-inflammatory drugs, antacid interactions, and anti-infective rashes accounted for 88% (143 of 161) of the adverse reactions and interactions. A number of adverse drug reactions and interactions were preventable in that careful attention to the patient's complete history, problem list, and relative to absolute contraindications to drugs should have resulted in drug changes or discontinuances in at least 61% (98 of 161) of the cases. An adverse reaction rate of 9.3% (161 of 1,728) of drug regimen reviews was found.

DEFINITIONS

Adverse drug reaction (ADR) is defined as any undesirable effect of drug therapy. Drug-drug interaction is a combination of drugs that may result in a beneficial or detrimental effect. For purposes of the study, only drug interactions of a detrimental nature were considered. Chapter 5 discussed drug contraindications or the presence of some condition or historical fact in the patient that indicates that a drug should probably not or absolutely not be used in the patient. This chapter discusses the development of undesirable consequences when the prescriber, pharmacist, and those administering the drug may not have been aware of these historical events or predisposing conditions, and adverse events occurred. Patients and responsible parties should be aware that ADRs are a common occurrence, be watching for these problems, and be informed when they occur.

Table 6-1 lists the types of adverse reactions and interactions encountered and the drugs involved in those DRPs. For purposes of this study, only those adverse reactions and interactions of possible to probable significance (i.e., some change had occurred in the patient that could be attributed to the drug) and moderate to major severity (i.e., change in drug indicated to problem of immediate to life-threatening nature) were included in the data reported.

The concept of preventable drug reactions must receive due attention. At least 61% of the documented ADRs could conceivably have been prevented by careful attention to the patient's complete problem list, including past ADRs, lab and physical findings, relative to absolutely contraindicated drugs, and the complete history of the patient. For example, a history of extreme sedation in a patient taking Mellaril® 25 mg TID need not be repeated when the patient is again placed on Mellaril® 50 mg BID. Another patient with renal impairment who was placed on a potassium-sparing diuretic and had a history of hyperkalemia when placed on the identical drug one year before had the identical hyperkalemia problem develop when the diuretic was restarted.

ADR-RELATED HOSPITALIZATIONS

A sample of six cases of ADRs that resulted in hospitalizations (CNS depression, hypotension, digoxin toxicity, GI bleeding [2 cases], and ampicillin anaphylactic reaction) were analyzed for estimated costs, for an average of $3,479 per episode. Assuming all 98 preventable ADR episodes could have resulted in hospitalizations, up to $340,942 of ADR treatment costs could have been avoided by careful attention to patient histories and known contraindications. At the point that the ADRs were detected and corrective recommendations made, 47 of the ADRs had resulted in hospitalizations. There could have been projected savings of $163,513 if careful at-

Table 6-1

Adverse Drug Reactions and Interactions in a 72-Bed Nursing Home
Over a 2-Year Period.

Drug Class(es)	Associated With Problem:	Number (%)	
Neurotropic			
Antipsychotics	Psuedodementia or	Single	
Anticonvulsants	CNS depression	Drug	16
Antianxiety agents	which improved on		
Antidepressants	discontinuance	Multiple	
Sedative/Hypnotics	(D/C) or drugs(s)	Drugs	19
Antihistamines	or lower dose		
and Opiate Analgesics		Sub-Total 35	(21.7)
	Low Blood Pressure		
Antihypertensive	Less than 110-120/60-70	Single	
Multiple Antihyperten-		Drug	23
sive(s)	Which increased on D/C	Multiple	
	of drug or lower drug	Drug	4
	dose	Sub-Total 27	(16.8)
K-Wasting Diuretic	Hyperkalemia	4	
with KCl Supplement	(K > 5.0mEq/L		
K-Sparing Diuretic	Hyperkalemia		
with KCl Supplement	(K > 5.0mEq/L	9	
K-Sparing Diuretic	Hyperkalemia	5	
without KCl Supplement	(K > 5.0mEq/L		
		Sub-Total 18 (11.2)	
K-Wasting Diuretic	Hypokalemia	11	
without KCl Supplement	(K < 3.5mEq/L		
		2	
with KCl Supplement	(K < 3.5mEq/L		
		Sub-total 13	

TABLE 6-1 (continued)

Drug Class(es)	Associated With Problem:	Number (%)
Digoxin Without Diuretic	Digoxin Toxicity Trough level > 2.0ng/ml chronic weight (1-2 lbs/ month) loss-poor appetite or pulse < 60 BPM 3 or more times per month which improved on D/C or	12
Digoxin Without Diuretic	lower dose drug	5
		Sub-Total 17 (10.6)
Nonsteroidal Antiinflammatory Drugs (NSAIDs)	Gastrointestinal Bleeding, positive occult blood in stool and/or decreased hemoglobin/hematocrit	Single Drug 16 Multiple NSAIDs 3
		Sub-Total 19 (11.8)
Antacids with Methenamine, Tetra- cycline, Iron Salts, or Digoxin	Patient infection anemia or heart failure not improved or worsened	8
		Sub-Total 8 (5.0)
Antiinfectives (Peni- cillins and Sulfonamides)	Allergic Rash	8 (5.0)
Antidiabetics	FBS Less Than 60 mg%	5 (3.2)
KCl Liquid and Anti- infectives	Diarrhea	2 (1.2)
Psylliuim Seed	Impactions due to insufficient oral fluids	1 (0.6) 1 (0.6)
Acetazolamide	Systemic Acidosis	1 (0.6)
Clindamycin	Pseudomembramous Colitis	1 (0.6)
Quinidine	Thrombocytopenic Purpura	1 (0.6)
Phenylbutazone/	GI ulcer perforation	1 (0.6)

Drug Class(es)	Associated With Problem:	Number (%)
Warfarin	and massive intrabdom-inal hemorrhage (Protime rose from 21.4 to 61 seconds).	
Opthalmic Dexa-methasone Drops (Continous)	Glaucoma/Cataracts	1 (0.6)
Nitrofurantoin	Hemolytic anemia, improved on D/C	1 (0.6)
Nitrofurantoin	Pneumonitis, improved on D/C	1 (0.6)
L-DOPA/Pyridoxine	Worsening Parkinsonism	1 (0.6)
	Total	161(100.0)

tention had been given to prior events and conditions in these patients. No attempt was made to determine drug-related mortality in this study.

It should be emphasized that the ADR events reported are episodes and that a number of patients had multiple episodes of ADRs. Specifically, 53 patients had 2 ADRs and 21 patients had 3 or more ADRs. Specific class reactions and interactions with case examples serve to illustrate ADRs.

NEUROTROPIC ADRs

The most frequent ADR was associated with antipsychotic medications (20 of 35 cases) given for control of the patient who had generally become uncontrollable and was endangering himself, fellow patients, and/or staff. Mellaril® was the most commonly involved single agent, followed by Navane® and Haldol®. The use of chemical restraints is not rational and must not be used for the patient who is disruptive rather than dangerous. Nevertheless, the practice does occur and can lead past the problem of excessive sedation to the problems of stasis-bedsores, pneumonitis, deep-vein thrombosis, constipation, and osteoporosis.

Multiple drugs were more often involved in excessive sedation and psuedodementia problems, as the following case demonstrates. An 84-year-old white female whose husband had died a month previously was given Valium® 2 mg prn sedation. After 12 to 15 doses over a 2-week period, she could not sleep and would complain to nursing staff. An order for Dalmane® was started, and within a week of nightly use, the patient developed acute brain syndrome with disorientation to time, place, and person; incontinence; and combative behavior. Mellaril® was started, and within three days, the patient was extremely sedated and had three decubitus ulcers. On discontinuance of all medications, the patient's mentation and functional capabilities were restored.

Further neurotropic ADRs concerned anticonvulsants (all Dilantin®), sedating antidepressants (Elavil®/Endep® and Sinequan®/Adapin®), and antihistamines when added to the regimen of a patient already on sedating medication(s).

ANTIHYPERTENSIVE ADRs

The Framingham studies clearly indicates that low blood pressure (BP) can be as detrimental as high blood pressure and can predispose to angina and transient ischemic attacks and confusion, as well as lead to heart attacks and strokes. Further problems of worsened orthostatic hypotension (precipitous fall in BP on arising) can lead to falls and fractures. The drugs most commonly involved in this problem were diuretics, followed by Aldomet® and Inderal®. The repeated finding of BPs less than 100-120 mm Hg systolic and 60-70 mm Hg diastolic mandates reevaluation of all medications known to affect blood pressure, including cardiovascular and psychotropic medications.

POTASSIUM BALANCE ADRs

The most likely event leading to these problems was failure to adequately monitor serum electrolytes (sodium, potassium, chloride, and bicarbonate) and renal function (serum creatinine). A baseline serum electrolytes should be established before a diuretic or potassium supplement is started and at least once after 30 days of therapy. Potassium is the most lethal drug in the acute care setting, and it must be carefully followed in the long-term care facility. Typical problems with potassium were the patient on Maxzide®, Dyazide®, or Moduretic® who had a potassium supplement or, in more recent years, ACE enzyme inhibitor (Capoten®, Vasotec®, Prinivil®/Vesprin®) started without a follow-up check of potassium status. Since all three diuretics — Maxzide®, Dyazide®, and Moduretic® — tend to conserve potassium, KCl supplements should be started very cautiously, if at all, and only after the diuretic combination present in these three agents has led to clinical hypokalemia. The same precautions hold when Capoten® or Vasotec® is started in the patient already on Maxzide®, Dyazide®, or Moduretic® or a diuretic plus potassium supplement. In terms of renal function, any patient with a serum creatinine greater than 1.5 mg/dl (normal = 0.5-1.5 mg/dl) should have more frequent monitoring of serum electrolytes, especially if potassium supplements or potassium-retaining products (which are relatively contraindicated) are to be used.

DIGOXIN ADRs

As may be seen in Table 6-1, digoxin toxicity may be seen with and without concurrent use of diuretics. The presence of hypokalemia (serum K less than 4.0 mEq/l) increases the likelihood of digoxin toxicity; conversely, the presence of hyperkalemia (serum K greater than 5.0 mEq/l) also predisposes to digoxin toxicity. Again, the monitoring of digoxin and electrolytes is an important factor in the prevention of toxicity. A trough level of 1.5 ng/ml or greater suggests the possibility of digoxin toxicity, most commonly manifested as anorexia with weight loss. On the other hand, digoxin has been discontinued in up to three-quarters of LTCF patients, especially when the patient does not have chronic heart failure or is in normal sinus rhythm and has a trough digoxin level of less than 0.6 ng/ml. At least 6 of 17 cases were being considered for hospital admission and work-up when digoxin toxicity was detected. Four cases had already been hospitalized for digoxin toxicity when detected.

NSAID ADRs

It is becoming clear that the NSAI given chronically to LTCF patients eventually lead to anemia in at least half of exposures and acute gastrointestinal (GI) bleeding in many cases. All NSAI (Motrin®, Clinoril®, Naprosyn®, Feldene®) in use, as well as ASA, were involved in these problems. In ten of these cases the patients had previously experienced GI bleeding. In all cases, the regular monitoring of hemoglobin/hematocrit (H/H) status (i.e., decreases in H/H of one gram/dl or more) every 2 to 3 months could demonstrate those patients who should have their NSAI stopped or prophylactic hematinic and/or protective therapy (Carafate®) started. The key points to watch for are a history of chronic arthritis, prior peptic ulcer disease, hiatal hernia, diverticulosis, and/or GI bleeding history.

ANTACID INTERACTIONS

Antacids taken internally can produce a number of significant alterations in the therapeutic effect of drugs. In the cases of methenamine complex agents (Mandelamine®, Hiprex®/Urex®) the antacids or calcium supplements can produce a more alkaline urine, and the methenamine prodrug is not broken down to its active ingredient, formaldehyde, unless urine pH is less than 6. In the case of the tetracyclines, iron salts, and digoxin, the antacid binds these drugs and prevents their absorption and their intended therapeutic effect. In all cases, patients' infection, anemia, or heart failure were not helped until the antacid was rescheduled to at least one hour before or two hours after the drugs that the antacid could bind.

ALLERGIC RASHES

In six of the eight cases, the allergic rash was a newly identified problem. Unfortunately, in two cases, patients who were penicillin-allergic on prior exposure were given the synthetic penicillins, ampicillin and amoxicillin, with near fatal results.

ANTIDIABETIC REACTIONS

All cases of antidiabetic reactions except one involved the use of insulin. The other case involved Diabinese®. Optimal control of older, Type II (maturity-onset) diabetic patients' fasting blood sugars (FBS) is probably 120-160 mg/dl. It is very dangerous to attempt to more rigidly control FBS, as many LTCF patients from time to time refuse to adhere to diet. In the cases detected, skipping meals more than likely contributed to all problems of hypoglycemia. It is of further interest to note that one of the patients was taking a beta blocker (Inderal®) that masked her hypoglycemic signs and symptoms, so the only way her low blood sugar could be detected was by her lab finding.

OTHER CASE FINDINGS

The other cases indicated in the table are all previously known reactions or interactions, with associated factors indicated in tabular fashion. This article has summarized perhaps the most serious drug-related problems in nursing home patients: adverse drug reactions and interactions. Through publication of these results, it is hoped that each nursing administrator, director of nursing, consultant/provider pharmacist, and medical director, as well as attending physician, will gain insight into ADR problems and will develop an ongoing program for prevention and detection of these problems before they occur. The consultant pharmacist's monthly report should reflect the ADRs detected or that could be prevented; it represents a currently required document that could be used for ADR surveillance and intervention purposes.[1] A checklist for ADRs is found in Figure 6-1.

Figure 6-1

A Checklist for Adverse Drug Reaction Detection, Prevention and Resolution.

1. Does the patient receive more than 3 regularly scheduled drugs ?

2. Has the patients condition deteriorated since the addition of any drug?

3. Can the attending physician justify each medication ordered?

4. Are doses of neuroactive drugs held due to oversedation, falls, daytime drowsiness ?

5. Have "drug holidays" been attempted in the patient with beneficial results ?

6. Do the patient and /or family/responsible party members understand why each drug is ordered?

7. Does the pharmacist routinely check each patients meds, their doses, and recommend changes in therapy ?

8. Do all nurses understand why each drug is ordered in the patient.

9. Can nurses tell what effect from a drug would prompt them to hold the drug for the patients safety?

10. Do the physicians and the medical director constantly try to reduce all meds and doses to the lowest number?

11. Does the administrator know the legal consequences of allowing chemical restraints to be used in patients?

REFERENCE

1. Cooper JW. Drug-related problems in a geriatric long term care facility. *J Ger Drug Therapy* 1986; 1(1):47-68.

Chapter 7

Nutritional Problems in a Geriatric Long-Term Care Facility

SUMMARY. Nutritional problems were the fourth most common drug-related problem encountered in a two-year study of DRPs in a geriatric LTCF. Nutritional problems were detected in 128 cases over 1,728 patient-care months and accounted for 10.5% of all DRPs. In descending order, problems encountered were weight loss, chronic infection, anemia, trauma or fracture, osteoporosis, serum albumin less than 3.5 g/dl or total lymphocyte count (TLC) less than 1500 without nutritional supplements, vitamins/minerals being given, and excessive weight gain. Implications of this study suggest that larger-scale nutritional studies should be conducted; the effects of nutritional intervention need further evaluation on clinical, moral, and ethical bases; and nursing homes perhaps need more definitive policy statements regarding the nutritional therapy of their patients.[1]

INTRODUCTION

The drug-related problems regarding nutritional considerations have not been detailed in long-term studies to date. A longitudinal length of stay study of nutritional changes in nursing home patients has been conducted recently.[2] One-fourth of the patients had severe malnutrition, either on admission or during their nursing home stay. Almost one-half of the patients either were anemic on admission or became anemic during their stay. The purpose of this study was to characterize and document the extent and types of nutrition-associated DRPs that occurred in a 72-bed geriatric LTCF over a two-year period.

METHODS

Nutritional DRPs were defined as any omission of needed therapy, when a patient exhibited physical, laboratory, or radiologic evidence of a problem that could be treated with nutritional therapy. In addition, any overuse of nutritional therapy or failure to restrict the diet when indicated by prudent therapeutic judgment was also considered a nutritional DRP. Patient chart review and physical and laboratory assessment and interpretation by a consultant pharmacist included a written problem list, evaluation of therapeutic goal attainment, and written communication to the director of nursing and attending physician.

DEFINITIONS

Nutritional problems were operationally defined as the patient with

1. consistent undesirable weight loss, with or without prior caloric restriction (e.g., diabetic);
2. inability or unwillingness to eat or poor appetite;
3. chronic infection;
4. anemia, with hemoglobin less than 12 g/dl in either sex, trauma, decubitus ulcer, or fracture;
5. laboratory values of serum albumin less than 3.5 g/dl, TLC less than 1500 (resting, not during acute infection), or hemoglobin/hematocrit less than 12/36;
6. insufficient caloric amount or intake or lack of multiple vitamin and appropriate minerals (iron for blood loss or iron deficiency anemias, zinc for wound healing, or calcium for osteoporosis and related fractures) to ensure positive nitrogen balance and weight maintenance or gain as appropriate.

Conversely, the patient whose lab values exceeded therapeutic goal (e.g., hemoglobin greater than 14 g/dl); whose weight had attained or exceeded prior "usual" or "ideal" weight; whose decubitus ulcer or fracture was healed or chronic infection was not present; or who did not show therapeutic response of improvement in weight, healing, or lab parameters despite nutritional therapy was considered to need reevaluation of nutritional/hematinic therapy.

All patients had monthly weighings and every one to three months had complete blood counts and chemistries conducted. All patients had monthly drug regimen reviews performed by their consultant pharmacists, with written comments on each patient reviewed and signed-off by the attending physician and the director of nurses coordinating any ordered changes in therapy. A consultant dietician was employed by the facility and was routinely informed of the consultant pharmacist's recommendations by review of the consultant pharmacist's monthly report.

RESULTS AND CASE ILLUSTRATIONS

The results are depicted in Table 7-1. Physicians accepted consultant recommendations in 93 of 128 cases (72.7%). Perhaps the best way to demonstrate the significance of these findings is via specific cases.

Weight Loss

A 79-year-old white female, 5'6", weighing 78 pounds, whose usual weight was 125 to 135 pounds, was taking digoxin 0.25 mg, with a trough level of 2.8 ng/ml (therapeutic levels are usually 0.6-1.5 ng/ml troughs) and taking Ritalin® 10 mg BID. She complained of no appetite and had lost 43 pounds over her 27-month nursing home stay. The consultant recommended discontinuance of her digoxin and Ritalin® (a potent appetite suppressant) and starting of multiple vitamins, one tablet BID, supplemental milkshakes with each meal, and dietary aides to be sure that she ate all food on her tray. Recommendations were accepted, and over the next 6 months she gained 21 pounds, had no problem with heart failure, and resumed knitting and interest in social activities in the facility.

Trauma

A 72-year-old black male with a history of prostate cancer, diabetes (adult-onset), and increasing disorientation over the last 3 months (since his wife died) had orders that included a 1200 calorie

Table 7-1

Nutritional/Hematinic Consideration‡

Problem	Number (%) of Problems	
Weight Loss (Without Nutritional Supplement, Vitamin or Appetite "Stimulant"	37	(29.8)
Chronic Infection, Anemia, Trauma, or Fracture (Without Nutritional Supplement, Vitamins, or Minerals)	29	(23.4)
Significant Osteoporosis Noted on X-Ray (Without Supplement Calcium Vitamin D Order)	18	(14.5)
Serum Albumin less than 3.5 Gm/dL (20) or Total Lymphocyte Count Less Than 1500 (4), With no Nutritional Supplement, Vitamins or Minerals)	12	(9.7)
Excessive Weight Gain (on Multiple Vitamins and/or Nutritional Supplement)	5	(3.9)
Problem no Longer Present	3	(2.3)
No Response to Recommended Treatment	3	(2.3)
	128	(100.0)

‡   See Operational Definitions App.A Ch.2

ADA diet, Valium® 10 mg TID prn anxiety started when his wife died, and Orinase® 500 mg BID. He was 5'11", 145 pounds, with 23 pounds weight loss over the past 3 months. During the past month he developed 3 decubitus ulcers, slept 12 to 18 hours per day, and was awakened with great difficulty. The consultant pharmacist recommended discontinuance of his Valium® and Orinase® (FBS = 68 mg/dl) and starting Stresstabs® with Zinc BID until the decubitus ulcer healed, with supplemental milkshakes BID and antacid/povidone iodine to the ulcers BID until healed. Within six weeks all ulcers (which ranged from Stage II to III) were healed, the patient had regained 15 pounds, and he was discharged to his daughter's home.

Osteoporosis

A 79-year-old, thin, frail white female with a history of wrist and hip fractures over the past three years was the victim of osteoporosis. On this month's review, an X-ray report done for suspected pneumonia revealed significant osteoporosis. This was noted, and calcium 1500 mg per day was recommended as 500 mg with each meal to ensure absorption. The recommendation was accepted and the calcium started. Within three days, the patient complained of constipation and gas and refused to take the calcium tablets. On discussion with the patient, a comprise was reached to start milk of magnesia 30 ml every other night for her constipation and simethicone 40 mg QID for her gas. After trying this regimen for two weeks, the patient again refused her calcium and stopped all medications. Conjugated estrogens 0.3 mg per day for three weeks on and one week off monthly were then recommended and accepted by both patient and prescriber, with limited acceptance of dairy products.

Nutritional Lab Abnormalities

A 62-year-old black female, 5'2", 267 pounds, with serum albumin of 2.8 g/dl (N = 3.5-4.5 g/dl) and TLC of 1100 cells (N = 1500-1800) had consumed a carbohydrate-predominant diet for most of her life and had recently developed adult-onset diabetes mellitus. She had been placed on an 800 calorie ADA diet but refused to comply with this spartan regimen. A recommendation of multiple vitamins, one tablet per day, with a 1400 calorie ADA was made, with grudging acceptance by the patient. A stroke ensued the next month, and the patient, who could not cheat by visits to the snack machines in the facility, lost 97 pounds over the next 2 years, with an increased percentage of her ADA devoted to vegetable protein and only complex carbohydrates (no sugar — only pasta, grains, or bread). Her serum albumin increased to 3.4 g/dl and TLC ranged from 1200-2100.

Excessive Response to Nutritional Therapy

An 84-year-old white female with hypothyroidism (treated) and underweight (5'4", 88 pounds) on admission to the facility was started on multiple vitamins along with Periactin® 4 mg TID to stimulate her appetite, and diet as requested. Within 6 months, her weight had increased by 41 pounds, and she had reached 158 pounds after a year in residence. At this time, her multiple vitamin and Periactin® were stopped, and the patient was put on a 1600 calorie per day dietary restriction. At the end of the next six-month period, her weight was stabilized at 132-137 pounds.

IMPLICATIONS OF RESULTS

This study did not routinely involve vigorous use of enteral or parenteral nutrition. There were many patients who were under "no code" orders and could be considered incapable of feeding themselves. If they refused dietary aid assistance, no attempt was made to "force-feed" or hydrate any patient. Over one-fourth of the recommendations were not accepted by the attending physicians, and this was accepted by the consultant. Ethical, moral, and legal questions regarding the physician's responsibility to the hopelessly ill patient have been reviewed.[3] This study illustrates some of the nutritional problems detected by a consultant pharmacist, who worked with the consultant dietician to improve nutritional therapy where feasible.

The use of a checklist for nutritional status evaluation is important for health care practitioners and patients and their families. Please see Figure 7-1 for a checklist.

Figure 7-1

CHECKLIST FOR NUTRITIONAL ASSESSMENT

1. Is the patient at their usual weight_____ lost weight _____?

    If weight loss is unintended, is this due to:

    a. poor dentition_____

    b. unable to feed self_____/ no interest in food____?

    c. aides not feeding patient_____

    d. poor food quality_____taste____ temperature_____ ?

2. Is poor nutrition and gradual starvation accepted by family or responsible party_____physician_____nurses_____ dietician_____consultant pharmacist_____?

3. If poor nutrition is not acceptable, have multiple vitamins and supplemental feedings been tried_____?

4. Are any of the following present (all necessitate improved nutrition) decubitus_____osteoporosis_____fracture_____ recent cold/flu/pneumonia_____low lab values_____?

REFERENCES

1. Cooper JW. Drug-related problems in a geriatric long term care facility. *J Ger Drug Ther* 1986; 1:47-68.

2. Cooper JW, Cobb HH. Geriatric nursing home patient nutritional changes during length of stay. *Nutr Supp Serv* 1988; 8(8):5-7.

3. Wanzer SH, et al. The physician's responsibility toward hopelessly ill patients. *New Engl J Med* 1984; 310:955-959.

Chapter 8

Nursing Home Drug and Nutritional Therapy Cost Savings

SUMMARY. This chapter presents cost savings to patients, their families, and the facility brought by vigorous consultant pharmacist services in one facility over a two-year period. Where patients or their families were unable to pay for medications or where their six prescriptions per month limit under Georgia Medicaid had been used, the recommendation of therapeutic alternatives, less expensive alternatives, and the use of routine house stock brought substantial savings to patient, family, facility, and Medicaid program. The recommendation of Medicaid formulary items when nonformulary items were prescribed was also well accepted by the prescriber. Cost savings from using combination products as opposed to single drugs were also evident.

INTRODUCTION

Previous chapters have demonstrated the detection, prevention, and consequences of drug-related problems in nursing home patients. The reduction of adverse drug reactions and subsequent cost savings were shown to be at least $186,000 to the health care system over a 2-year period. A prior study in this facility found a quantitative reduction of over $32,000 per annum when the consultant was employed and a doubling of drug costs per year when the consultant was not employed.[1] This chapter presents the cost savings that resulted when the qualitative aspects of drug and nutritional therapy were pursued over a two-year period.

The objectives of this study were to:

1. Evaluate existing drug and nutritional therapy for potential areas of therapeutic substitution that could result in cost savings to the patient and family;
2. Recommend therapeutic substitution or alternative therapy to the attending physician;
3. Follow patient acceptance and therapeutic benefit of accepted recommendations; and
4. Compile recommendation acceptance, outcome, and cost changes.

Methodology

The methods employed in this study were:

1. Rigorous drug regimen review that involved
   a. Writing a problem list after a thorough review of the patient's chart and all pertinent data, as well as physical assessment of the patient;
   b. Matching all therapy with a problem or indicating where there was therapy with no apparent problem;
   c. Evaluation of therapeutic need, goal attainment, and drug toxcicity;
   d. Assessment of potential therapeutic alternatives which, if substituted for the original therapy, could save costs to any of the parties involved;
   e. Communication of significant therapeutic substitution recommendations to the attending physician of the patient.
2. Team conference with charge nurses, director of nursing, social worker, dietician, and attending physician, when available, for discussion of total patient therapy, patient and family acceptance and/or complaints regarding costs of therapy;
3. Discussion with patient and/or the family regarding total therapeutic plan and cost-effectiveness of alternatives to existing therapy.

Drug and nutritional therapy costs were computed based on actual acquisition cost or average wholesale price from the 1984 Redbook plus the professional fee allowed by the Georgia Medicaid program at the time of this study. Costs were defined as expenditure of resources by any party involved in the payment of health care costs.

RESULTS

The results of therapeutic alternative substitution recommendations are listed in Table 8-1. This data was originally reported without cost analysis as a type of drug-related problem.[2] Case examples serve to illustrate the bases for therapeutic alternative recommendations.

Acetaminophen or Enteric-Coated Aspirin for NSAID

An 85-year-old white female Medicaid patient with osteoarthritis, diabetes mellitus, high blood pressure, constipation, malnutrition, and peripheral vascular disease routinely exceeded her six prescription per month limit and had to use her $25 per month Medicaid personal expenditure allowance to pay for her medication. After discussion with the patient and attending physician of possible ways to decrease her drug costs, her medications were cut from seven regular schedule and three as needed medications to seven total medications, and acetaminophen 650 mg QID was substituted for her naproxen 375 mg BID, which had been costing her $30 to $35 per month. Her regular schedule acetaminophen (APAP) cost $8 to $10 per month and produced relief of her arthritic pain similar to the naproxen. Furthermore, her propoxyphene napsylate with acetaminophen as needed medication, which she had been using several times a week, was stopped once regular schedule acetaminophen was started.

An earlier study has demonstrated that regular schedule acetaminophen is superior to narcotic-aspirin or narcotic-acetaminophen combinations given on an as needed basis, both in terms of analgesic effect and overall drug administration costs.[3] Similar patient situations where enteric-coated aspirin (ECASA) was preferable to acetaminophen (e.g., pain with inflammation or

Table 8-1

Drug and Nutritional Therapy Recommendations

Problem	Recommendation	Number(% of problems)
Patient/Family Unable to pay for med and/or 6 Rx/month limit reached*	Acetaminophen for NSAID**	12 (9.7)
	Enteric-coated ASA for NSAID	18 (14.5)
	Whole milk/milkshake for enteral feeding supplement	29 (23.4)
	Less expensive Alternative	37 (29.8)
Rx not on Medicaid Formulary	Recommendation of formulary:	
	Laxative	9 (7.3)
	Hematinic	6 (4.8)
	Therapeutic Multiple Vitamin	8 (6.5)
Single Drugs used together in same patient on a regular schedule basis	Conversion of single drugs to combinations (e.g. Aldoril, Apresazide, Inderide, Maxzide)	5 (4.0)

total 124 (100.0)

*Over 90% of patients in this study were medicaid-covered. Georgia medicaid reimbursement is limited to 6 prescriptions per month.

post-myocardial infarction or stroke patients), produced similar efficacy and patient acceptance and showed similar cost savings. A prior study conducted when nonsteroidal anti-inflammatory drugs (NSAIDs) were taken off the Georgia Medicaid formulary showed ECASA to be as effective as NSAIDs at a much lower cost.[4] An important difference between APAP and ECASA is that the latter is covered by Medicaid, but APAP is not on the Georgia (or many other states') Medicaid drug list. The difference is that APAP would have to be paid for by the patient where floor stock is not used or allowed by regulation. This is, perhaps, a mistake in that when NSAIDs cause anemia or an acute gastrointestinal bleed, APAP is clearly the safer choice for relief of noninflammatory arthritic pain. Based on an average cost to the patient of $4.68 per month for APAP, compared with an average cost of $33.52 per month for the NSAID, the 12 patients were saved an average of over $4,100 per year of pain therapy. In the case of ECASA, the Georgia Medicaid system was saved, based on an average ECASA cost of $6.05 per month versus the NSAID average cost of $33.52, almost $6,000 per year for the 18 patients switched from NSAID to ECASA.

Whole Milk/Milk Shakes for Enteral Feeding Supplements

An 88-year-old black male, 5'11", weighing 116 pounds, with diagnoses of prostate cancer and malnutrition had lost 47 pounds in the 6 months prior to admission to the facility. His orders included liberal diet, Ensure® one can TID as a supplement, DES 25 mg per day and multiple vitamins one BID. He objected to the taste of the feeding supplement and, despite the use of flavor packets, repeatedly refused to take the supplement. On the consultant pharmacist's assessment and recommendation, the patient was switched to milk shakes TID, which was well accepted by the patient. Over the next 6 months, the patient gained 23 pounds, and his serum albumin rose from 3.2 to 3.8 g/dl. Based on a cost to the facility of $0.92 per 8 oz. can compared with $0.08 per 8 oz. serving of whole milk and $0.13 per 8 oz. whole milk and 4 oz. ice cream added, the 29 patients switched from enteral feeding supplements to whole milk or milk shakes saved the facility between $25,000 and $27,000 per year in feeding supplement costs. The claimed advantage of many enteral feeding supplements is that many nursing home patients are lactose-intolerant. A standing order for lactase enzyme, 2 drops to be added to the milk or milk shake 10 minutes before administration, was not needed in any of the 29 patients. Two patients preferred the enteral feeding supplement they had been on and were switched back to that product.

Less Expensive Alternative Therapy

There were several areas where less expensive therapeutic alternatives were recommended with varying degrees of acceptance and therapeutic success. Salt substitutes packets were recommended for 21 patients requiring potassium chloride supplements with their potassium-wasting diuretics. The recommendation was accepted in 10 patients, but none was successfully converted for more than a month. The reasons for poor conversion were that the salt substitutes were not reliably measured or given, as bulk or as packets. The most economical way to conserve potassium levels in the patient who needs this conservation is by the use of potassium-wasting and sparing diuretic combinations (e.g., Maxzide®, Moduretic®, Dyazide®) in place of the diuretic and potassium chloride solid or liquid dosage form therapy. In fact, this use of combination therapy has been shown in a prior study to save almost $10 per month compared with the cost of the 2 separate prescriptions.[5]

Conversion to Medicaid
Formulary-Covered Medications

The conversion of patients to formulary listed laxatives, hematinics, and vitamin products saved the 19 patients in 28 episodes a total of $2,290 per year. All recommendations were accepted by the attending physician.

Conversion to Combination Products

In the five cases where patients were converted to combination products, the annual cost savings to the state Medicaid system was $465.60 over the cost of both prescriptions.

SYNOPSIS AND CHECKLIST

This chapter has demonstrated areas where consultant pharmacists' recommendations, when requested by patient/family or facility and accepted by the attending physician, can produce substantial drug cost reduction to the patient, facility, and Medicaid reimbursement system. A checklist of important questions to raise concerning drug therapy costs and alternatives is given in Figure 8-1.

Figure 8-1

CHECKLIST FOR DRUG COST SAVINGS

1. Has a thorough drug regimen review been conducted_____?

2. Are all drugs prescribed necessary for the patient_____?

3. Are generic and therapeutic equivalents being used_____?

4. Are less expensive drugs available_____?

5. Are combination products being used where feasible_____?

6. Do my physician and pharmacist seem willing to discuss this issue?

REFERENCES

1. Cooper JW. Effect of initiation, termination, and reintitiation of consultant pharmacist services in a geriatric long term care facility. *Med Care* 1985; 23:84-86.

2. Cooper JW. Drug-related problems in geriatric long term care facility patients. *J Ger Drug Ther* 1986; 1:47-68.

3. Wilcher DE, Cooper JW. Consultant pharmacist effect on analgesic/anti-inflammatory usage in a geriatric long term care facility. *J Am Ger Soc* 1981; 29:429-432.

4. Spruill WJ, Cooper JW. Enteric-coated aspirin efficacy in patients previously treated with non-steroidal anti-inflammatory agents. *South Med J* 1983; 76:27.

5. Cooper JW. Efficacy and cost-effectiveness of a new diuretic-combination in a geriatric long term care facility. *Curr Ther Res* 1986; 39:160-165.

Chapter 9

Reduction of Irrational Drug Duplication in Geriatric Nursing Homes

SUMMARY. The reduction of irrational drugs and duplication by rigorous drug regimen review, in-service education, and physician acceptance of consultant pharmacist recommendations in a geriatric long-term care facility is described. In decreasing order of frequency of duplication, laxatives, analgesics, NSAIDS, diuretics, hypnotics, antipsychotics, KCl supplements, hematinics/vitamins, antacids and antinauseant and antidiarrheals were the drug classes most often duplicated. Apparent reasons for the duplications were confusion over the term, "_____ of choice," physician convenience, failure to actively review medication orders, and individual nurse preferences for different agents in each duplicated drug class.

INTRODUCTION AND METHODS

Previous chapters describing drug-related problems in long-term care facilities have documented reduction of medication errors, drug contraindication and adverse reaction, nutritional deficits, overall drug costs and drug-related hospitalizations and mortality detected by the consultant pharmacist. The purpose of this chapter is to document the types of drug duplication found on rigorous drug regimen review and to determine the apparent reasons for these duplications.

The objectives were to:

1. Write a complete problem list after thorough chart review (problems included established diagnoses; physical, psychological, or physiological abnormality; abnormal sign/symptom or lab test; noncompliance by patient, prescriber, or nursing

staff; past operations and adverse drug reactions). A copy of this problem list was placed in the front of each patients chart;
2. Match all therapeutic modalities (drug, dietary, etc.) with the problem(s) when logical (recognizing that some drugs may not relate to an active problem and that some problems may not have been assessed or treated) on a monthly basis;
3. Identify drug use patterns for all agents (i.e., were all ordered drugs being used as ordered) on a monthly basis;
4. List drug duplications deemed unnecessary by rational therapeutic knowledge and standard pharmacotherapeutic references;
5. Communicate therapeutic change recommendations to the prescriber on a monthly basis; and
6. Tabulate recommendation acceptance rates and postulate reasons for the duplications.

RESULTS

The results are indicated in Table 9-1. The attending physician accepted 51 of the 78 recommendations (65.4%) as previously noted.[1] Further breakdowns of the frequency of each drug and the types of duplications are found within the individual drug class sections, along with an illustrative case.

Laxatives

The 20 cases involved an average of 3 laxatives per patient. The most frequently prescribed type of laxative was the irritant type, with or without a stool softener (e.g., Dulcolax®, Ex-Lax®, Doxidan®). In view of the recent removal of danthron-containing products and earlier studies linking chronic irritant cathartic use with lower bowel cancer, it would seem imprudent to use this type of laxative in any patient. Mineral oil was also commonly prescribed, despite its association with the development of lipid pneumonia with chronic use. Bulk laxatives, (e.g., Metamucil®) and stool softeners (e.g., Colace® and Surfak®) were also commonly prescribed. Despite the standard recommendation that bulk laxatives be used in sufficient quantity to make the stools "float," a relative underdos-

Table 9-1

Irrational Drug Duplication

Therapeutic Class	Number(%)
Multiple:	
Laxatives	20 (25.6)
Analgesics	16 (20.5)
NSAIDs	10 (12.8)
Diuretics	8 (10.3)
Hypnotics	6 (7.7)
Antipsychotics	6 (7.7)
KCl supplements	4 (5.1)
Hematinics/vitamins	4 (5.1)
Antacids	2 (2.2)
Antinauseants/Antidiarrheals	2 (2.6)
Total	78 (100.0)

ing was noted, with the average dose being less than a tablespoonful. The prn use of stool softeners is not effective, yet they were commonly prescribed, ". . . as needed." Lactulose and sorbitol were not routinely prescribed. Milk of magnesia (MOM) was the second most common prn laxative. In a recent five-year study of chronic constipation in nursing home patients, MOM given on a regular basis, in doses ranging from 30 ml every third night to 60 ml nightly, was found to be the most effective laxative for preventing impactions and enema use.[2] A representative case history serves to demonstrate the multifaceted nature of this problem.

An 87-year-old female with chronic regular schedule medications of Lasix® 40 mg/day, Elavil® 50 mg HS, Motrin® 400 mg QID and FeSO$_4$ 325 mg TID PC and prn medications to include MOM 30 ml prn, ASA 5 grs q 4 h prn, DSS 100 mg prn, Metamucil® 5 ml prn, Dulcolax® suppositories prn, and SS enemas was noted to have had 2 impactions during the previous month. Several doses of each laxative were used. Nurses stated that the patient drank only small amounts of fluids and refused her Metamucil®. The consultant recommended discontinuance of her DSS, Dulcolax® and Metamucil® and a regular schedule of MOM 30 ml every other night. When this recommendation was accepted by both prescriber and patient, no further impactions were noted over a three-month period. On referral to this patient's admission orders, the order ". . . laxative of choice," was noted. The question must be raised whose choice is to be followed, the nurse(s) or the patient's? On questioning each nurse who had received the order for each laxative, it was found that each drug was her personal choice, and the prescriber simply added each order at each nurse's request. An in-service was given at the 7-3 and 3-11 shift change on appropriate laxative use, the importance of adequate fluid intake, and more careful monitoring of bowel function when diuretics, psychotropics, iron salts, and NSAIDs are added to the patient's regimen.

Analgesics

Multiple analgesics were the second most common duplication. The failure to adequately review orders and to combine orders for the single analgesics aspirin and acetaminophen were the reasons for these duplications. A propoxyphene plus acetaminophen compound (e.g., Darvocet®-N 100) was the most commonly used prn pain medication, followed by a barbiturate plus aspirin (e.g., Fiorinal®). In the 16 cases of irrational duplication, patients were receiving an average of almost 2.5 analgesics, with 1 or more doses per month. (NOTE: This facility had a stop order policy that any drug not given once during a 60-day period could be automatically discontinued.) A further reason for the apparent duplication of drugs with analgesic activity was the writing of one drug (e.g., aspirin for ". . . fever or aches") and another for pain (e.g., acetaminophen). An earlier study has documented that when a prn pain medication, either single or combination product, is given on a basis of at least twice daily, the therapeutic substitution of regular schedule acetaminophen 650 mg 3 to 4 times a day is more efficacious for pain relief.[3] This also saves 8 to 10 hours per 100 patient beds per week in nurses' time accounting for prn drug effect and schedule drug reconciliation.

An 81-year-old black male with osteoarthritis, depression, and constipation had medication orders (doses in last month) including Darvocet®-N-100 (14), Axotal® (24), ECASA 10 grs (23), Tylenol®

(33) (all prn) and Norpramin® 50 mg HS and MOM 30 cc prn constipation. The consultant pharmacist recommendation was to put Tylenol® on a 650 mg QID regular dose basis and discontinue Darvocet®, Axotal®, and ECASA the next month if no doses were used. All three extra analgesics were subsequently stopped, and Tylenol® stayed on a regular schedule. An in-service on pain control was given, and a protocol for all drug requests to go through the director of nursing was instituted.

Non-Steroidal Anti-Inflammatory Drugs (NSAIDs)

NSAIDs were duplicated in ten patients. The primary duplication concerned a regular schedule of NSAIDs such as Motrin®, Clinoril®, Tolectin®, Feldene®, Naprosyn®, or Meclomen® with a prn dose of ASA or ECASA. This is not only irrational, but if used together these drugs can increase the risk of significant GI bleeding at least three to four fold over the use of either agent alone. Some rheumatologic authorities prefer the combined use of these two agents, if the risk is justified. In seven of the ten cases, a subtherapeutic dose of the NSAID was being used. In three cases, a regular schedule of two NSAIDs was being used. In the two cases where the attending physician refused to alter this regimen, both patients were hospitalized with significant GI bleeding within six months after the second NSAID was started. A recent study found that a significant proportion of nursing home patients receiving regular schedule NSAIDs became anemic within three to six months after their NSAID was started.[4] Therapeutic substitution of acetaminophen or ECASA 650 mg QID for the NSAIDs is as effective as previously noted and is unlikely to cause significant GI blood loss, unlike ASA or the other NSAIDs.

A 71-year-old white female with chronic multiple-site pain complaints had orders for Feldene® 20 mg per day, ASA 10 grs q 4 h prn aches or pains, $FeSO_4$ 325 mg BID, and Mepergan Fortis® one q 6 h prn severe pain. She received several doses of both ASA and Mepergan® per week and became progressively disoriented and anemic over a two-month period. On the consultant pharmacist's recommendation, the Feldene®, ASA, and Mepergan Fortis® were stopped and ECASA 10 grs QID started, with better control of pain complaints. Similar findings were noted in 43 of 45 patients who were converted from newer NSAIDs to ECASA.[5] The patient's mental status improved over the next month, and her iron therapy was also stopped, as her hemoglobin increased 2.0 g/dl from 10.3 to 12.3 g/dl after the Feldene® and ASA were stopped. The Demerol® in the Mepergan Fortis® causes significant disorientation, as do Talwin® and Darvocet®. Such disorientation can lead to acute brain syndrome or pseudodementia, mimicking Alzheimer's disease. Narcotic analgesics containing propoxyphene were the second most common (to Valium®/Dalmane® type medications) drugs causing adverse reaction on admission to a nursing home.[6]

Diuretics

Diuretics are prescribed for the control of high blood pressure and congestive heart failure. Eight patients were receiving diuretics in the same therapeutic class (thiazides in seven cases and loop-type in the eighth). The apparent reasons for the duplication were use of less than maximal dose of the first diuretic prescribed, decreased bioavailability of the diuretic prescribed first, physician lack of knowledge that both combination products prescribed had diuretics as one of the components, and failure of the physician to review the orders. Specifically, in respective order, physician ordered Maxzide® to be added to the regimen of a patient already on hydrochlorothiazide (HCTZ) 25 mg per day when an increase in the HCTZ or simply changing to Maxzide® alone would have been more rational. Dyazide® formerly had bioavailability problems (since corrected, according to verbal communications with company sources), causing three patients to have HCTZ added as a second diuretic to their regimen. Two patients had two combination products containing diuretics, Ser-Ap-Es® and Dyazide®, and Minizide® and Combipres®, both of which have thiazide diuretics. One patient had prn orders for both HCTZ and Lasix® ". . . as needed for edema." This patient had borderline congestive heart failure and consistent blood pressures above 160/90 mm Hg and needed a regular dose of HCTZ for her CHF and HBP. The final patient's physician had prescribed both Lasix® and Bumex® (both are potent loop diuretics) for CHF and needed simply to increase the dose of Lasix®, rather than add a second diuretic.

A pharmacotherapeutic note regarding the use of diuretics from different classes is important. It is rational therapy to use both a thiazide (e.g., HCTZ) and a loop (e.g., Lasix®) in the same patient, as each diuretic works on a different part of the nephron. Similarly, it is quite rational to use both a potassium-wasting (e.g., HCTZ) and a potassium-sparing diuretic (e.g., triamterene or amiloride) in the same combination product (e.g., Dyazide®, Maxzide®, or Moduretic®).

Hypnotics

The use of hypnotics for more than 7 to 14 days on a daily basis is not rational drug use. Furthermore, the chronic use of the longer acting benzodiazepines (e.g., Dalmane®) is commonly associated with acute brain syndrome when given on a daily basis, especially when 30 mg strength is used. All six patients in this study had more than one sleep medication and used one or more doses per month (e.g., Dalmane® prn and Restoril® prn). Only two of six cases had the duplicated medications discontinued. The nurses who requested their favorite hypnotic were resistant to having their orders stopped. A prior study of hypnotic use found that most of the chronic use was irrational, and the underlying problem was probably depression, requiring the use of antidepressants.[6]

Antipsychotics

Antipsychotics were the drugs most frequently implicated in adverse drug reactions in nursing home patients. The apparent reasons for the duplication of these agents were that the prescriber wrote for use of the different drugs for symptoms such as ". . . agitation, restlessness, sedation, aggression, calming, etc." on separate occasions, usually at the nurse's or facility's request, and did not review or cancel previous orders for other psychotropic medications. The result was that the patient could receive as many as four psychotropic drugs in the same month. It should be realized that all psychotropic drugs can cause psuedopsychiatric problems of drug-induced dementia, depression, and oversedation. Oversedation itself leads to the stasis problems of bedsores, pneumonia, constipation, deep vein thrombosis, and faster osteoporosis. In all cases, two of which required family member intervention with the physician, the duplications were stopped and more rational approaches to assessment of psychiatric problems employed. A typical case follows.

A 77-year-old white female whose husband had died three months prior to her admission was found wandering in a rural field by her children 2 weeks after her Valium® Rx to help her over her husband's death was started. She was admitted to a nursing home with admission diagnosis of chronic brain syndrome or Alzheimer's disease, and Mellaril® 25 mg tid and 75 mg HS were started. Within a week the patient was more agitated, and Navane® was added ". . . prn agitation." The next week, after ten Navane® doses, the patient was not improved, and Haldol® ". . . prn restlessness" was added. All throughout this period, the patient's Valium^R was continued. After nurse and family discussions, the consultant recommended discontinuation of all psychotropics, which was grudgingly accepted by the prescriber only after family insistence. Within a two-month period the patient markedly improved; oriented to time, place, and person; was able to resume care of herself; and was discharged.

It may not be assumed that all psychotropic drugs are irrational in nursing homes, but an earlier study in a similar home found that over two-thirds of psychotropics could be stopped, with improved patient mentation and alertness the usual result.[6]

Potassium Supplements

The duplication of potassium supplements in all four cases involved the routine use of liquid KCl or solid KCl (e.g., Slow-K®) with salt substitutes (e.g., Co-Salt®). In three of the four cases, the patient had potassium levels above 5.0 mEq/l (normal serum K = 3.5-5.0 mEq/l), and the salt substitute was ordered as part of a dietary sodium restriction. The last case involved the patient's family bringing in the salt substitute without prescriber approval, and the patient's serum potassium was 6.5 mEq/l and pulses were less than 50 BPM. As recently noted, potassium can be the most lethal drug given to patients.[7]

Hematinics/Vitamins

This duplication was noted when patients were both malnourished and anemic. Two of the cases involved use of both a hematinic (e.g., Trinsicon®) and a therapeutic multiple vitamin/mineral with many of the same vitamins and minerals. Two of the cases were the use of two hematinics in possible anemia of senescent patients, whose hemoglobins and hematocrit levels would not increase over 10 g/dl and 30, respectively.

Antacids, Antinauseants, and Antidiarrheals

In all cases of duplication of drug classes, it appeared that the attending physician had failed to realize or review his orders, and the drugs were irrationally used. Again, in-service on proper antacid use, the significance of nausea and diarrhea, and the drugs for these conditions was given after the orders were discontinued.

IMPLICATIONS AND CHECKLIST

This chapter has documented typical drug duplications found over a two-year period in a nursing home. Rigorous drug regimen review, nurse vigilance to drug effect, and regular in-service reduced irrational duplication, and these may be viable methods to improve rational drug therapy in the long-term care facility. A checklist can serve to detect and prevent needless drug duplication. Please see Figure 9-1.

Figure 9-1

DRUG DUPLICATION CHECKLIST

1. Is there more than one drug given regularly for each verified patient problem_____?

2. Are there multiple orders for symptoms , rather than diagnoses, such as pain, agitation/restlessness/nervousness_____?

3. Is the physician willing to present the basis for all drugs_____?

FIGURE 9-1 (continued)

```
4. Will the pharmacist tell me which drugs are not life-saving_____?

5. Are there many "...as needed..." orders which are never used_____?

6. Are there any drugs which could be used for more than one diagnosis?

7. Are there any drug combinations that could save on prescriptions__?
```

REFERENCES

1. Cooper JW. Drug-related problems in a geriatric long term care facility. *J Ger Drug Ther* 1986; 1:47-68.

2. Cooper JW. Chronic constipation in the geriatric nursing home patient—a five year study. *J Pharmacoepid* 1990 1(2).

3. Wilcher DW, Cooper JW. Consultant pharmacist effect on analgesic/antiinflammatory usage in a geriatric long-term care facility *J Am Ger Soc* 1981; 29:429-432.

4. Cooper, JW, Mallet L, Wade WE. Anemia detection, treatment and outcomes in a geriatric long term care facility. *J Pharmacoepid* 1(1):61-70.

5. Spruill WJ, Cooper JW. Enteric-coated aspirin efficacy in patients previously treated with NSAIDs. *South Med J* 1983; 76:276.

6. Cooper JW, Francisco GE. Psychotropic drug usage in long term care facility patients. *Hosp Form* 1981; 16:407-419.

7. Miller, RR, Greenblatt, DJ. Drug effects in hospitalized patients. John Wiley, New York, 1976.

Chapter 10

Questionable Drug Efficacy in Dementia, Anemia, and Urinary Infections

SUMMARY. Drugs ordered on a chronic basis for patients of a skilled nursing facility were reviewed for efficacy as part of drug regimen reviews over a two-year period. Drugs classified as "less than effective" or "probably ineffective" by the National Academy of Science/Drug Review Council (NAS/DRC) findings and clinical judgment as well as established clinical practice literature were questioned in 47 episodes: papaverine in dementia (25); multiple vitamin/tonic without iron in iron deficiency or blood loss anemia (8); methenamine complexes in chronic urinary tract infections (CUTI) where the patient was catheterized, had a urine pH greater than 7 and/or had consistent urinalyses indicating 4 + bacteria while on the drug (6); trimethoprim/sulfamethoxazole (5) or nitrofurantoin (2) in patients with CUTI and consistent urinalyses with 4 + bacteria; and oral hematinic with vitamin B_{12} in a patient with documented pernicious anemia. The attending physician accepted recommendations for discontinuance or change of these inefficacious medications in 42 of 47 episodes for an acceptance rate of 89.4%. In no cases of discontinuance was a worsening of patient dementia or an increase in frequency of UTIs noted. All patients with anemia had improved hematologic findings on change to an efficacious agent. Nursing home administrators, physicians, medical directors, nurses, directors of nursing, and pharmacists should not hesitate to question the use of drugs they believe are not of benefit to the patient. This type of drug-related problem has many facets related to the quality of patient care in nursing homes.

INTRODUCTION

Earlier chapters have discussed the drug-related problems (DRPs) of medication errors, relative contraindications to drug use, adverse drug reactions and interactions, nutritional/hematinic problems, socioeconomic problems with drug use and irrational drug duplication. The purpose of the study presented in this chapter was to examine the use of drugs with questionable efficacy in geriatric nursing home patients.

METHODS

The methods used in this study and the demographics of this population have been published previously.[1] For brief review, this was a population with a mean age of 81 years, 90% female, with an average of over three established diagnoses and slightly over six drugs per patient (regular and prn schedule with monthly doses). Rigorous monthly drug regimen reviews were conducted monthly on each patient by a doctoral-level consultant pharmacist with tabulation of pertinent recommendations on each patient by the attending physician via a manual list. The director of nursing was responsible for attempting to coordinate total therapy and recommendations to the respective attending physicians, including the recommendations of a consultant dietician, a social worker, a physical therapist, and a pharmacist.

The operational definitions of questionable drug efficacy were established by the National Academy of Sciences/Drug Review Council (NAS/DRC) classification of a drug as ''less than effective'' or ''probably ineffective'' in a standard reference, such as the *Physicians Desk Reference (PDR)* or the *United States Pharmacopoeia Dispensing Information (USPDI)*, American Hospital Formulary Service (AHFS), or Applied Therapeutics, or primary articles on pharmacotherapy from the published reputable literature. The input of the charge nurse was sought regarding the purported efficacy of the drug in question in cases where a subjective impression was necessary. For example, the question was raised in the case of the use of papaverine in dementia as to whether any subjective improvement in patient condition, mentation, or capability for activities of daily living was observed by the charge nurse, nursing supervisor, or director of nursing, both before the recommendation for discontinuance was made and after the discontinuance. In the case where an objective observation could be made (e.g., number of documented UTIs or the hemoglobin/hematocrit readings both before and after the order change), such observations were re-corded.

Cost-savings from the order change recommendations were cal-culated using average wholesale price of the drug per the 1984 Redbook plus the dispensing fee of $4 per prescription.

RESULTS

The results of questionable drug efficacy findings are indicated in Table 10-1. Case or case data compilations serve to illustrate indi-vidual detection and management techniques. Papaverine generi-cally or in any of its trade name forms (Pavabid®, Vasal®) has never been shown to be of benefit in dementia or in the poststroke patient. In fact, this drug and a number of others purported to be of benefit

Table 10-1

Questionable Drug Efficacy in Dementia, Anemia and Presumed Chronic

Urinary Tract Infection

Questionable Drug Class	Condition	Number(%)	
Papaverine	Dementia	25	(53.2)
Multiple Vitamin tablet/ tonic/elixir without iron or sub-therapeutic iron	Iron deficiency or blood loss anemia	8	(17.0)
Methenamine complexes in catheterized patients with urine pH greater than 7, and consistent 4+ bacteruria	Presumed Chronic Urinary tract Infection(CUTI)	6	(12.8)
Trimethoprim/Sulfamethoxazole or nitrofurantoin in CUTI pateient with 4+ bacteruria	CUTI	7	(14.9)
Trinsicon	Documented Pernicious Anemia	1	(2.1)
	total	47	(100.0)

in Alzheimer's or other dementias or poststroke care, such as cyclandelate (Cyclospasmol®), isoxsuprine (Vasodilan®), nylidrin (Arlidin®), and Hydergine®/Trigot®/Decapril®, are no longer on the Medicaid reimbursement list of approved drugs because of the lack of demonstrated efficacy of these agents.

A 77-year-old black female with a history of high blood pressure, stroke, and moderate dementia had orders for hydrochlorothiazide 12.5 mg per day, Pavabid HP® one bid, and diet ad lib. Her right-sided hemiplegia and inability to speak despite poststroke physical and speech therapy hindered her assessment, but the charge nurses continually responsible for her care stated that they had seen no improvement in her mentation; affect; or disorientation to time, place, and person since her stroke and the start of Pavabid®. They further believed that she was not so demented as to classify her as "moderate," but they believed that her inability to communicate had contributed to her lack of desire to stay oriented to time, place, and person. All lab work was within normal limits, and her blood pressure was 112/68-136/78 for the prior three months. After her physician accepted the recommendation for discontinuance, her three-month assessment found little change, except that her blood pressure ranged from 116/72-140/86 for that period. In 22 of 25 cases, the papaverine was stopped with no change in patient condition. The projected cost savings to the patient, as the Medicaid-eligible patients could not get this unapproved drug paid for, was $85 per average patient year or 22 × $85/pt. = $1,870 per year for the facility.

In all eight episodes of iron deficiency or blood loss anemia, the physician believed that the patient's multiple vitamin tablets or tonic/elixir also contained a therapeutic amount of iron (which they did not). On conversion to a therapeutic oral iron product, all eight patients' hemoglobins/hematocrits (Hgb/Hct), which had been below an acceptable value of 12/36 (before = 10.5/33.2 average), were above 12/36 after 3 months of appropriate iron therapy (after = 12.5/37.8 average). There was negligible cost change on the average when patients were switched to a therapeutic iron preparation.

Methenamine complexes (Mandelamine®, Hiprex®/Urex®) are intended to release formaldehyde in the bladder of patients whose urine pH is 6 or below, thereby sterilizing the urine and preventing colonization of bacteria which could lead to an acute infection. In the catheterized patient, the collection bag becomes the bladder, making methenamine complex agents useless. Furthermore, most patients which chronic urinary tract infections (CUTIs) have recurrent Proteus species involved in their infections, especially if they also have a history of kidney stones. Proteus, Pseudomonas, and some Staph species make a urease enzyme that cleaves urine urea and other nitrogenous substances into ammonia, producing basic urine pHs (above 7). This further contributes to methenamine lack of efficacy. Finally, most nursing home patients also have an alkaline-ash diet (primarily dairy products, vegetables, low in protein) that contributes to an alkaline urine. Add to this the fact that a number of drugs also alkalinize the urine (e.g., antacids, calcium supplements, thiazide, and CAI diuretics), and one can note that the methenamine products have little chance of helping to prevent the occurrence of UTIs in the nursing home patient. In the six patients, who had an average of 1.8 treated UTIs in the 3 months before methenamine discontinuance, a slight drop in UTI frequency was noted (1.2 UTI/patient) over the next 3 months. The number of observations was too small to treat statistically, so the possibility that this change in UTI frequency was due to chance alone cannot be excluded. No other agents, such as those below, were substituted for the methenamine agent that was discontinued. The savings to the Medicaid reimbursement system averaged $187 per patient year.

Just as methenamine complexes have not been shown to affect the frequency of UTIs in nursing home patients with CUTI (usually defined as two or more infections every six months), neither have trimethoprim/sulfamethoxazole (TMP/SMX, Septra®/Bactrim®) nor nitrofurantoin (NTF, Furadantin®/Macrodantin®) been shown to decrease UTI frequency. The physicians denied recommendations in two of seven cases. In those five patients who had either agent stopped, there was no change in UTI frequency three months before and after the agent was stopped (average number of UTIs before = 3.1/pt.; after = 3.0/pt.). The finding of 4+ bacteria in all CUTI patients, despite therapy, more than likely reflects a colonization due to a natural or instrumented (catheter) incontinence, where the continual urine stream leak provides a pathway for mobility of the bacteria from the introitus/meatal area up the urethra into the bladder. In all cases, there appeared to be treatment of urinalyses rather than patients. Simply put, a routine urinalysis was ordered on each patient receiving prophylactic anti-infective therapy. When a finding of 4+ bacteria was phoned into the physician's office, usually with a concomitant urinalysis finding of occasional white blood cells (wbcs), it was assumed that the patient was symptomatic and thus needed an antibiotic. For this reason, routine urinalyses are not recommended in the patient capable of complaints, unless the charge nurse also observes significant symptoms or signs (e.g., change in urine smell) that may indicate significant infection. Otherwise, the routine ordering of antimicrobials for asymptomatic bacteruria will be the rule. Unfortunately, the use of anti-infectives for the asymptomatic patient will result in bacterial resistance to the usual oral anti-infectives, necessitating the use of more expensive oral or injectable agents for the next infection, which inevitably occurs.

The questionable efficacy of the drugs used to treat CUTIs has two parts: (1) the use of chronic drugs that do not work for prophylaxsis which, in the case to TMP/SMX and NTF, added an average of \$292 per patient year and (2) the use of other anti-infectives, at an average of \$53 per pseudoepisode for an average waste of \$636 per patient year. Attempts to change prescribing behavior in the second part were unsuccessful. The further question of making patients more susceptible to resistant infections, which may prove fatal if they lead to Gram-negative sepsis, was not explored in this study.

The one case of documented pernicious anemia in which an oral B_{12} agent was being used with no improvement in megaloblastic anemia was changed to B_{12} injection with subsequent improvement in hematologic picture. If patients develop pernicious anemia, they usually do so because they have developed antibodies to their own gastric intrinsic factor, which is needed for the absorption of dietary B_{12}. The use of oral hematinic preparations that contain animal intrinsic factor usually results in the body making cross-antibodies to the animal intrinsic factor within weeks after the start of the oral agent. This makes the oral B_{12} ineffective and mandates the use of injectable B_{12} in any patient with documented pernicious anemia.

IMPLICATIONS

This chapter presents a study regarding the use of inefficacious drug therapy in nursing home patients demonstrating that a number of drug prescribing habits for dementia, anemia, and presumed chronic urinary infections produce less than optimal patient care and unnecessary drug expense. It is presumed that all nursing home administrators, directors of nursing, and pharmacists are cognizant of the consequences of questionable drug prescribing as illustrated in this study and that they have action plans to reduce this type of drug-related problem. A practical list of questions to address this issue is found in Figure 10-1, a checklist for questionable drug prescribing.

Figure 10-1

A Checklist for Questionable Drug Presribing and Efficacy

1. Are all the drugs prescribed helping the problem they are intended to treat_____?

2. If a drug has not been shown to improve a condition, why is it being used_____?

3. Are all drugs prescribed on the Medicaid-reimbursement list_____?

(If a drug or dosage form is not on this list, it is highly likely that either the drug is not effective, or there are less expensive drugs that are therapeutically equivalent and available or covered)

REFERENCE

1. Cooper JW. Drug-related problems in geriatric nursing home patients. *J Geriatr Drug Ther* 1986; 1(1): 47-68.

Chapter 11

Lack of Recognition and Treatment of Active Problems in Geriatric Nursing Home Patients

SUMMARY. The underrecognition and lack of treatment of active problems in a nursing home over a two-year period of time were studied. Forty-seven cases of therapeutic need without treatment or dosage schedule change needed were identified via a problem list, intensive drug regimen review, and physical and lab assessment of patients by a consultant pharmacist. In decreasing order (cases), need to treat high blood pressure (13), obstipation (10), symptomatic urinary tract infection (5), hypokalemia (4), osteoarthritic joint pain (4), chronic endogenous depression (4), glaucoma by history (2), persistent angina pectoris (2), seizure activity (2) and transient ischemic attacks (TIAs) (1) were brought to the attention of the six attending physicians. In 40 of 47 cases (85%), the physician accepted the therapeutic recommendation of the consultant pharmacist. Refusal to treat seven of the cases identified involved high blood pressure (3) and one case each of depression, angina, seizures, and TIAs. Quality of care considerations and legal responsibilities are reviewed.

INTRODUCTION AND PURPOSE

Prior chapters have dealt with the improper use of drugs in nursing homes detected by rigorous drug regimen reviews conducted by a consultant pharmacist.[1] The purpose of the study presented in this chapter is to document how adequately patient problems were assessed and treated in a nursing home over a two-year period.

METHODS

The patients in residence within this facility received an initial workup, with problem list, matching of therapy with problems, and assessment of therapeutic goal attainment and communication of significant drug-related problems to the attending physicians through the director of nursing on a monthly basis, as mandated by the 1974 federal mandate for the consultant pharmacist to "monitor the drug regimen of the patient on a monthly basis. . . ." Significant problems of underrecognition, underdiagnosis, and undertreatment were classified as such when standard treatment guidelines in accepted reference materials were not followed. Furthermore, the professional knowledge of treatment standards resulting from the consultant pharmacist's prior professional responsibilities for coordinating and teaching in both baccalaureate- and doctoral-level therapeutics courses were used in determination of therapeutic inappropriateness.

RESULTS

The results of the therapeutic recommendations made over the two-year study period may be noted in Table 11-1. Presentation of illustrative cases with each category and reasons for the inappropriate treatment noted serve to focus the attention of nursing home administrators and directors of nursing, medical, and pharmacy services on methods to detect and solve these problems in their facilities.

High Blood Pressure

The established blood pressure at which some form of regular treatment should begin is defined by the National High Blood Pressure Coordinating Committee as between 140/90 and 160/95 mm Hg. Such readings found on three or more consecutive occasions, preferably a week apart, dictate that dietary restriction of sodium to two grams per day, weight-loss and caloric restriction if obesity is present, and graded exercise program if possible be undertaken before pharmacologic intervention is begun.

Table 11-1

Therapeutic Need but No Treatment Ordered for Exisiting Problem

Problem	Recommendation	Number (%)
High Blood Pressure	Initiate low-dose diuretic or vaso- dilator therapy	13 (27.7)
Obstipation/Impaction	Regular Schedule MOM plus increased oral fluids	10 (21.3)
Urinary Tract Infection	Appropriate antiinfective	5 (10.6)
Hypokalemia	KCL supplement or K- sparing diuretic in combination product	4 (8.5)
Osteoarthitis	Regular schedule acetaminophen	4 (8.5)
Chronic depression	desipramine	4 (8.5)
Glaucoma	timolol eye drops	2 (4.3)
Persistent angina pectoris	regular topical NTG	2 (4.3)
Seizure activity	phenobarbital	2 (4.3)
Transient ischemic attacks	ASA 325mg/day	1 (2.1)
		47 (100.0)

An 82-year-old 5'4", 186-pound, white female with a history of high blood pressure, one prior mild heart attack, angina pectoris, and atrial fibrillation had orders including regular diet ad lib, Apresoline® 25 mg po prn BP greater than 190/100, Trans-Derm® nitro-5 one patch daily, Lanoxin® 0.125 mg daily, NTG 0.4 mg SL prn, MOM 30 ml hs prn, and ECASA 10 grs q 4 h prn aches, pains or fever. Her blood pressures for the month had all exceeded the 140/90 to 160/95 limit, but only on 3 occasions had her pressures met the order guidelines to give Apresoline® doses. She did have persistent headaches over this period and received 26 doses of ECASA. Her attending physician believed that her "normal" systolic blood pressure should be 100 plus her age, and he declined to order regular treatment of her HBP. She had been "doing fine with that BP for a long time, and he didn't want to make her fuzzy-headed by lowering a brain perfusion pressure she had grown accustomed to over the years." The patient experienced a fatal stroke during the next month, and her death was attributed to "natural causes." The Framingham studies have clearly shown that systolic blood pressures over 140 mm Hg are the clearest prognostic indicator for the risk of stroke. While there is controversy over what level to begin treatment with drugs, there are convincing results, such as the European Working Party study, of the reduction of stroke and heart attack risk by appropriate treatment and lowering of BP to levels below 140/90 mm Hg.

More than half of the high blood pressure seen in nursing home patients is of the isolated systolic type, in that systolic pressures are consistently over 160, with diastolics less than 90 mm Hg. Again, while the clear-cut benefits of pharmacotherapy have not been unequivocally demonstrated, it is known that failure to treat these elevated systolics and to reduce pressures to below 140-160 mm Hg is the main proximal cause of morbid cardiovascular and cerebrovascular events. The fear of making patients less coherent because of lowering their elevated BP is answered very simply: gradual lowering of HBP over several weeks is preferable to allowing the patient to suffer from failure to adequately treat the high blood pressure. During a period of several weeks after appropriate drug therapy is started, some initial disorientation and "fuzzy-headedness" may be evident, but once the baroreceptors reset after 10 to 14 days of gradual BP lowering, the patient becomes more lucid. On the other end of the HBP treatment spectrum, this problem may be overtreated. If BPs are consistently below 110/60 mm Hg, a dose reduction or elimination of HBP medications may be needed, as too low a perfusion pressure may also cause infarction of the heart and brain. All three cases not treated appropriately were due to physician insistence on letting BPs exceed 190 mm Hg before any treatment was given, and then only on the days that this pressure was exceeded could the drug be given. All three patients died of strokes within six months of entering the facility.

Obstipation/Impactions

Over one-half of 335 nursing home patients studied over a three-year period developed chronic constipation.[2] In this study ten cases of chronic constipation were found by noting the weekly or more frequent use of prn laxatives, such as milk of magnesia, and/or at least one use of an enema over a one-month period of time. In all cases, a combination of drug, patient, and facility factors contributed to the problem. Drugs likely to cause constipation include diuretics, NSAIDs, iron, zinc and calcium salts, and anticholinergic drugs, such as all psychotropics, antihistamines, some antiulcer drugs (e.g., Donnatal®, Robinul®, Pro-Banthine®, and some anti-incontinence drugs (e.g., Ditropan®). Patient factors included lack of sufficient fluid and food intake. Facility factors included lack of bowel retraining program and recognition of the need for attention to stool records. In the case of bowel retraining, the simple morning routine of giving the patient a warm beverage, placing the patient on the commode for 30 minutes, when coherent, and encouraging fluid intake throughout the day was needed. In the stool records, blank spaces and aides' failure to call a period of two to three days without a stool to the nurses' attention were noted. The validity of the stool records (i.e., some apparent falsifications were noted) is also a problem.

The removal of impactions or the patient having to strain to defecate are not only unpleasant but can be fatal, as the increased intrabdominal pressure created by the Valsalva maneuver (straining) or rectal distention to remove impactions can produce fatal cardiac arrhythmyias.

A 77-year-old male with HBP, osteoarthritis, suspected peptic ulcer disease, and mild constipation, had Lasix® 40 mg started one week. The next week, Feldene® was started for arthritic pains. Within a month, the Feldene® had caused stomach upset, and Donnatal® was started. Stool frequency decreased from daily to two to three stools a week, despite good food intake. After three enemas and eight doses of MOM were given during the next month, the consultant pharmacist recommended a regular schedule of MOM 30 ml every other night. On this schedule, no further enemas had to be given.

Urinary Tract Infections

The last chapter on questionable drug efficacy questioned the efficacy of chronic anti-infective therapy in patients with chronic urinary tract infections. In this study in the same population, five cases of failure to treat valid UTIs were found. The apparent reason for failure to treat patients with symptoms of dysuria, frequency, urgency, urine culture, and sensitivity of colony counts of bacteria greater than 100,000 per cubic mm was failure of follow-up from the physician's office when these problems were called in by the nursing home charge nurse. At the other extreme, many facilities irrationally use routine urinalyses (U/As). The reason that these U/As are irrational is that many physicians assume that because a result is called into their office, they must initiate treatment of the patient.

The fact is that virtually all patients with urinary incontinence will have U/As suggesting bacterial colonization, but this is not acute infection unless the coherent patient has symptoms of dysuria, frequency, or urgency in the case of lower UTI and these symptoms plus flank pain, fever, and chills in the case of both lower- and upper-tract UTI.

Hypokalemia

Four cases of hypokalemia (serum potassium less than 4.0 mEq/l), all due to the use of potassium-wasting diuretics (e.g., hydrochlorothiazide, furosemide) without potassium supplement or potassium-sparing agents (e.g., triamterene, amiloride, or spironolactone), were noted. In all cases, the physician did not believe that hypokalemia becomes significant until serum K is less than 3.0 mEq/l. Recent cardiac studies have found that serum K should be 4-5 mEq/l, whether the patient is on digitalis or not, to protect the heart from fatal hypokalemia-associated arrhythmias. Up to 60% of sudden deaths attributed to natural causes in patients taking potassium-depleting diuretics were, in fact, due to low total body potassium.

Osteoarthritis with Persistent Joint Pain

Patients should not have to suffer chronic pain without some chronic prophylactic analgesic therapy. Regular schedule acetaminophen, 650 mg QID in the patient with good liver function, is the safest way to anticipate pain and to reduce the prn irrational use of narcotic combinations that can confuse the patient and make him appear to be demented (e.g., Darvocet®-N 100, Wygesic®, Percodan®, Percocet®, Talwin® compound). In fact, 650 mg of acetaminophen or enteric-coated aspirin is superior to most of the above-mentioned narcotic combinations in that they all contain ASA or acetaminophen. Nonsteroidal agents (NSAIDs) are much more expensive and far more likely to cause significant anemia and GI bleeding than either acetaminophen or enteric-coated aspirin.

Chronic Depression

No patient wants to enter a nursing home. After an initial period of adjustment for situational depression, the chronic signs and symptoms of poor appetite, lack of interest or socialization or activities of daily living, even though they are capable, suggest depression. Additionally, up to one-third of those patients with definite dementia of the Alzheimer's type have concurrent depression as part of their problem. In three of the four cases, the attending physician ordered desipramine (Norpramin®/Pertofran®) 25 mg q AM the first month, with monthly increases of 25 mg, up to 100 mg daily. Also, chronic use of long-acting hypnotics or sedatives (e.g., Dalmane®, Valium®, Paxipam®, Centrax®, Tranxene®) was stopped in a further six patients, as chronic use of these agents can lead to a chronic drug-induced depression or dementia that is extremely difficult to treat with antidepressant therapy. These long-acting agents should probably be stopped after 7-14 days of use as sleepers or 3-4 months of daily use for anxiety to prevent the likelihood of drug-induced problems.

Glaucoma

All persons over age 40 should have an annual check of their intraocular pressure. In the two cases noted, the patients had a history of glaucoma before nursing home admission, but their glaucoma medications had inadvertently not been continued on admission.

Persistent Angina Pectoris

In one case a patient with chronic chest pains was being given nitroglycerin ointment "prn chest pain." Since it takes 30 minutes to an hour for the ointment or patch to release therapeutic amounts of NTG to the circulation, routine use of the ointment was recommended but denied by the attending physician. The patient died of an acute myocardial infarction in the professional judgment of the charge nurse, but the death certificate read natural causes.

Seizure Activity and Transient Ischemic Attacks

In three cases, these problems were continually observed and noted in the chart, but in only one case would the prescriber order effective prophylactic therapy.

IMPLICATIONS

The nursing home administrator and the directors of nursing, medical, and pharmacy services must maintain vigilance over the appropriate therapy of problems found in the facility. While these results are anecdotal in that they are from only one facility, the implications are clear: make sure patients are treated correctly or face the legal consequences. Patients and their responsible parties should question whether all active diagnoses are being treated, as in Figure 11-1.

Figure 11-1

A Checklist for Establishing Therapeutic Need Assessment

1. Are all patients problem lists complete and updated monthly by the nursing, physcian and pharmacy staffs?_____

2. Is the attending physician willing to discuss the rationale for each problem in each patient with the nursing and pharmacy staffs and patient/family/responsible party ?_____

3. Are there clearly defined treatment goals for each pharmacotherapeutically-treatable problem on the problem list of each patient?_____

4. For example are the goals are as follows:

a. High blood pressure- maintain BP at 120/70-140/90 mm Hg.

b. Angina pectoris-no attacks which may be perceivable.

c. Diabetes mellitus-FBS below 160, but no lower than 100 mg/dL.

d. Peptic ulcer disease, recurrent-no reoccurence of gastric pain/gastritis or anemia.

e. Anemia-hemaglobin >12 g/L in most, >10 g/L in anemia of senescence or chronic disease and > 8 g/dl in chronic severe renal failure.

REFERENCES

1. Cooper JW. Drug-related problems in geriatric nursing home patients. *J Ger Drug Ther* 1986; 1(1):47-68.

2. Cooper JW. Chronic constipation, drug and patient factors and prophylactic laxative efficacy. *J Pharmacoepidemiology* 1991; 1(2).

Chapter 12

Appropriate Use of Laboratory Tests in the Nursing Home

SUMMARY. The appropriate use of laboratory tests was studied by a consultant pharmacist in a geriatric nursing home over a two-year period. Over the study period, there was a general underuse of drug levels to detect digoxin, phenytoin, and theophylline effects and occasional underuse of serum electrolytes and serum creatinine to monitor diuretic effects and to determine appropriate use of drugs in renal impairment. Prescriber acceptance of 95% (40 of 42) of consultant pharmacist recommendations for lab monitoring brought changes in drug therapy with 35 of 40 cases (87.5%). Of 35 prescriber-authorized lab determinations, 32 (91.4%) resulted in significant results that changed drug therapy dose or schedule or necessitated additional therapy. The total cost of the requested lab work was $2,560 over the 2-year study period. On the other hand, the overuse of routine multiple lab tests on a monthly to bimonthly basis yielded new information in less than 5% of repeated determinations. Routine lab work that was in excess of the federal indicators frequency and situation recommendations produced $71,566 of excessive and, perhaps, unnecessary health care costs over this 2-year period.

INTRODUCTION

Prior chapters have focused on the areas of medication errors, relative contraindications and adverse reactions and interactions with drugs, nutritional assessment, socioeconomic considerations, drug duplication, questionable drug efficacy, and therapeutic need for drug therapy. The purpose of the study presented in this chapter was to document the therapeutic need for adequate laboratory tests to monitor and assess the effects of drug therapy in a geriatric long-term care facility over a two-year period.

Specific objectives were to:

1. Determine the clinical utility of selected lab tests for the assessment of drug effect;
2. Document the outcomes of both selected requested and routine lab determinations in geriatric nursing home patients;
3. Calculate the relative costs of selected versus routine lab tests; and
4. Evaluate the relative outcome efficiency of selected versus routine lab tests.

METHODS AND MATERIALS

All patients in a skilled nursing facility served by six physicians, eight provider pharmacists, and one consultant pharmacist were evaluated by intensive drug regimen review conducted by a doctoral- level consultant clinical pharmacist over a two-year period. On admission or initiation of consultant clinical services, each patient had a thorough chart review and intensive drug regimen review consisting of:

1. Writing a problem list of all present and past problems that could influence drug therapy outcome;
2. Matching of all therapeutic modalities with problems;
3. Assessment of patient physical and lab parameters needed to adequately evaluate therapeutic outcome in each patient via clinical judgment and established guidelines, such as the federal indicators and reference texts;[1,2]
4. Communication of significant suspected problems necessitating further lab assessment or requesting less frequent use of routine lab orders where there is no clinical basis, either pathophysiologic or pharmacologic, for the sustained use of the routine tests; and
5. Follow-up evaluation of levels ordered, refused to be done, or

done too frequently, for significant data essential to patient care.

The operational guidelines for drug levels were:

1. Clinical judgment was based on patient signs, symptoms, body weight, renal and hepatic function tests, if available. A trough level, taken just before the first dose of the day, was done rather than risking wasting money on other levels taken at some point on the approach or decline from maximum or peak levels.
2. Any interacting drugs (e.g., quinidine with digoxin, and cimetidine with theophylline or phenytoin) prompted a follow-up physical assessment of symptoms and estimated effect on any prior levels, whether actual or estimated. A repeat or initial level was ordered based on this clinical judgment.
3. A projection of peak effective level was made, and if higher trough levels that could go into toxic ranges or were uncorrected for serum binding were found, a written communication of this correction or projection was made to aid the prescriber in the interpretation of the drug level.

Other lab work determinations were made primarily on the basis of clinical judgment, with the minimal guidelines of the federal indicators and established long term care references.[1,2] For example, the indicators recommend: (indicates recommended change)

Drug Class/Agents	Test(s)	Frequency
Diuretics	Serum Electrolytes or Potassium	Within 30 days of initiation of diuretic therapy, dose increase or addition/deletion of potassium-affecting therapy. Repeat in 6 months
Diuretics and Digoxin	Ditto	Ditto

Drug Class/Agents	Test(s)	Frequency
Injectable Aminoglycosides/ Garamycin, Nebcin Amikin, Netromycin Kanamycin, Streptomycin	Serum Creatinine	Before and after Course of Treatment (if treatment is longer than 7 days, repeat every 7 days)
NSAIDs/Butazolidin Azolid (NOTE: THESE DRUGS ARE NOT RECOMMENDED AT ALL in the patient over 60 per FDA Bulletin 1985;14:23)	Complete Blood Count(CBC)	Within 30 days of therapy
Other NSAIDS/ Motrin,Feldene Orudis, Naprosyn Tolectin, ASA Disalcid, Trilisate Dolobid, Clinoril	Hemaglobin/Hematocrit (H/H)	Within 30 days of start(and every 60 days thereafter)
Hematinics/Iron/ folic acid/B12	Ditto	Ditto
Urinary Tract Antiinfectives for Prophylaxsis/ Mandelamine/Hiprex/ Urex/Septra/Bactrim	Urinalysis(U/As)	Within 30 days of start of therapy NOTE: ROUTINE U/As ARE NOT RECOMMEDNDED- as lab slips rather than patients tend to be treated.
Urinary Antiseptics/ Mandelamine/Hiprex/ Urex	Urine pH 6 or below	Within 30 days of start of therapy (and q 30 days).
Nitrofurantoin/	Serum Creatinine	Before or during first

Drug Class/Agents	Test(s)	Frequency
Macrodantin/Fura-dantin	or BUN	30 days of therapy
Insulin/Oral Hypoglycemics	Fasting Blood Sugar (FBS)	Before therapy started and every 30 days while on antidiabetics
Oral anticoagulant/warfarin/Coumadin	Prothrombin time (PT)	Before therapy and every 30 days while on anticoagulant.
Thyroid or Antithyroid agents	Thyroid Function Tests	Before therapy (and every 6 to 12 months while on therapy)
Anticonvulsants/Dilantin/Depakene Mysoline/Phenobarbital	Drug levels	When patients lose seizure control or appear toxic.

RESULTS

The results of this study are indicated in Tables 12-1, 12-2, and 12-3. Table 12-1 indicates that the selected request of lab tests to include drug levels, based on clinical judgment of a consultant pharmacist who performs both physical and laboratory assessment of the patient on a monthly basis as part of intensive drug regimen review, is reasonably efficient. In contrast, a recent study found that the use of routine digoxin and theophylline levels in a VA long-term care facility rarely influenced patient management, regardless of results. On the other hand, abnormal results of assays ordered for clinical indications resulted in patient management changes in about 50% of cases.[3]

The results in Table 12-2 point out that the routine frequent use of test batteries in the geriatric nursing home produces few new results that markedly change patient care. A recent study of the yield of annual laboratory tests in a skilled nursing home population found that 17% of tests gave abnormal results, with slightly over one-third

Table 12-1

Lab Test Needed to Assess Drug Therapeutic/Toxic Endpoint

Problem/Drug Class	Test Requested	Number:Requested	Done	Significant
Suspected Digoxin Toxicity/underdose	Trough Digoxin level	24	22	18(82%)
Suspected Hypo- or Hyperkalemia with Diuretics and/or KCl supplements	Serum Electrolytes	8	8	6(75%)
Suspected Renal Impairment with Nitrofurantoin/ aminoglycoside use	Serum Creatinine	4	4	4
Suspected Dilantin Toxicity	Dilantin/Serum Albumin levels (trough)	4	4	4

Table 12-1 Continued--

Suspected Theophylline Toxicity	Theophylline trough levels	2	2	2
	Totals (%)	42(100)	40(95)	35(88)

of these results being new data. Almost 17% of the abnormal results brought benefit to one-fourth of the patients studied.[4] It is of interest to note that in all cases in the present study population, the recommended frequency of lab testing was exceeded.[1] Table 12-3 presents possible excessive costs incurred in the study population, primarily by routine use of lab tests. The contrast between this study, with the use of almost monthly urinalyses, bimonthly CBCs, and quarterly SMAs, and the previously mentioned work is that in both studies about 1 in 20 tests/test batteries done resulted in patient benefit.[4]

SUMMARY AND CONCLUSIONS

This chapter shows that in one nursing home both judicious and excessive use of lab tests occurred. The main reason for the inefficient use of lab tests appeared to be exceeding the recommended indicators for drug monitoring and regimen review. While the

Table 12-2

Routine Lab Test Average Frequency and New Findings in 72-Bed LTCF

Test	Average Frequency Per/Patient/Year	New Findings From Test or Battery per Patient/Year
Complete Blood Count or H/H	6.3	0.23 (3.7%)
SMA 12	3.4	0.16 (4.7%)
Urinalysis	10.7	0.44 (4.1%)

Table 12-3

Cost Analysis of Lab Tests Ordered Over a Two-Year Period in a 72-bed Geriatric Nursing Home

Test	$ Cost	Significant Yield(%)	Possible Excessive Cost
Digoxin level	50	18/22 (82)	4x50=$200
Electrolytes	60	6/8 (75)	2x60=$120
Ser.Creatinine	16	4/4 (100)	-
Phenytoin	50	4/4 (100)	
Theophylline	50	4/4 (100)	
CBC	30	37/907 (3.7)	870x30=$26,100
SMA-12	46	23/490 (4.7)	467x46=$21,482
Urinalysis	16	62/1541(4.0)	1479x16-$23,664

total excess cost $71,566

present study cannot be assumed to be representative of all nursing homes' use of lab tests, the guidelines and results given may be useful to nursing home administrators, medical directors, attending physicians, directors of nursing, and pharmacists working in long-term facilities.

A checklist for monitoring appropriate use of lab tests appears in Figure 12-1.

Figure 12-1

A Checklist for Appropriate Lab Test Utilzation Asssessment

1. Are the tests as stated in methods, being conducted for the drugs being used in the patient_____?

2. Are Medicaid, Medicare or the Third-Party Insurance paying for these tests_____? If not, why not_____?

3. Does there appear to be over-or underutilization of lab tests for the patient(s)_____?

REFERENCES

1. Federal Indicators for Drug Regimen Review. Transmittal No. 174, DHHS, HCFA, State Operators Manual-Provider Certification.

2. Cooper JW. Drug therapy monitoring guidelines. Haworth Press, New York, 1990.

3. Silbergeit IL et al. Routine assays of serum levels of digoxin and theophylline in a long term care setting: essential monitoring or expensive fad? *J Ger Drug Ther* 1988; 3(1): 63-72.

4. Levinstein MR et al. Yield of routine annual laboratory tests in a skilled nursing home population. *JAMA* 1987; 258:1909-1915.

Chapter 13

Inappropriate Dosing Interval
and Drug Scheduling
in a Geriatric Nursing Home

SUMMARY. The inappropriate scheduling and administration of medications in a geriatric nursing home was studied by a consultant pharmacist in a geriatric nursing home over a two-year period. There were 24 documented cases of inappropriate drug scheduling noted. They concerned antibiotics (12) given with meals rather than before meals or being dosed over 4- rather than 8-hour intervals, antacids with meals and medications, rather than 1 to 2 hours after meals (6), and antipsychotics/antidepressants given 3 to 4 times a day or at inappropriate times (6). The primary reason for the scheduling errors was the lack of a central pharmacist who both dispensed and scheduled the medication orders. The use of modified unit-dose rather than eight separate pharmacies with an individual prescription system could have prevented virtually all of these inappropriate schedulings of drugs. A 100% compliance rate with the consultant pharmacist's recommended changes was noted.

INTRODUCTION

Previous chapters in this drug-related problem series have focused on medication errors, relative contraindications and adverse reactions and interactions with drugs, nutritional assessment, socio-economic considerations, drug duplication, questionable drug efficacy, therapeutic need for drug therapy, and appropriate use of lab tests. The purpose of this study was to assess the appropriateness of drug scheduling and administration by provider pharmacists and charge nurses in a geriatric long-term care facility over a two-year period.

111

Specific study objectives were to:

1. Determine the appropriate scheduling of medications from dispensing to administration and documentation in the medication administration record (MAR); and
2. Document the outcomes of inappropriate scheduling of drugs and follow-up on recommended scheduling changes.

METHODS AND MATERIALS

All patients in a skilled nursing facility served by six physicians, eight provider pharmacists, and one consultant pharmacist were evaluated by intensive monthly drug regimen review conducted by a doctoral-level consultant clinical pharmacist over a two-year period. On admission or initiation of consultant clinical services, each patient had a thorough chart review and intensive drug regimen review consisting of:

1. Writing a problem list of all present and past problems that could influence drug therapy outcome (kept in front of chart);
2. Matching of all therapeutic modalities with problems;
3. Assessment of patient physical and lab parameters needed to adequately evaluate therapeutic outcome in each patient via clinical judgment and established guidelines, such as the federal indicators and reference texts.[1,2]
4. Communication of significant suspected problems necessitating further scheduling of drugs and verifying that the recommended scheduling changes were made and documented to the charge nurse and director of nursing by review of original doctor's orders, MAR, and pharmacy profile.

The operational definitions for appropriate drug scheduling were:

1. All drugs known to have gastrointestinal irritant potential were to be given with or after meals (please see Table 13-1) in P.C. med passes.
2. All drugs that should be given before or away from meals or away from other drugs were to be scheduled to allow optimal

drug administration and to avoid inefficacious therapy (Table 13-2).

3. All drugs scheduled to give less than optimal therapeutic effect were to be rescheduled to promote more continuous levels of the medication or more appropriate timing of drug pharmacologic effect (see Table 13-3).

RESULTS AND DISCUSSION

The results of this study are indicated in Table 13-4. The practice of giving antibiotics with, rather than before, meals was the most common scheduling problem noted. In four of the eight cases, the antibiotic was ordered *ante cibos* (a.c.) but was actually written to be given with meals when transcribed from the doctor's order and

Table 13-1
Drugs/Classes Which Should be Given With Food or After Meals

Antihypertensives	Prednisone
Antidiabetics	Nitrates
Aspirin	NSAIDs(Motrin, Naprosyn,Clinoril,Tolectin
Atromid-S	Ansaid,Orudis,Naproxen, Feldene, Meclomen)
Azolid (Should not be used in those Over 60)	
Azulfidine	Pyridium
Chloral Hydrate	Reserpines
Deacdron	Salicylates
Dilantin	Theophyllines
Iron, Calcium, Potassium and Zinc Salts	
Flagyl	Multiple Vitamins
Fulvicin	Minerals of any type
Furadantin	Narcotics, oral
Grifulvin/Grisactin	Sulfas (Bactrim/Septra)
Indocin	Urecholine
INH	Zyloprim/Lopurin
L-Dopa (Dopar) and L-Dopa/carbidopa (Sinemet)	
Macrodantin	

prescription label. The most practical problem with giving antibiotics such as tetracyclines and erythromycins before meals is that they irritate the esophagus and stomach, especially when given with very little water. Many cases of esophageal ulceration have been reported when insufficient water is given with tetracycline capsules. The most obvious solution to this problem is to give the tetracycline capsule with two full eight-ten oz. glasses of water or other fluids, not the one to two ounce fluid cups used on many medication carts. If sufficient fluid cannot be given, then a request to change the dosage form to tetracycline or erythromycin liquid dosage form is justified to ensure absorption of the drug. Food with all tetracy-

Table 13-2

Drugs Which Should be Given Before or Well After (1-3 hrs.)

Meals to Prevent Problems of Absorption or to Allow for Maximal

Therapeutic Effect

Anticholinergics (for decreasing gastric secretions) Robinul, Donnatal

Pro-Banthine, Levsin, Daricon, Atropine

Antacids and Carafate

Antibiotics such as tetracyclines, erythromycins, Noroxin, Cipro

Antiulcer agents such as Tagamet, Zantac, Pepcid and Axid are best

given at bedtime on a once daily schedule, or with the start of a meal

if given more than once a day.

Table 13-3

Drugs which should be given over the period of a day when dosed BID or

TID

Drugs	Dosed As	Should be Given as
Antibiotics	BID	q 12 hours (7-7 to 10-10)
Eye meds, sustained action meds		
Antibiotics	TID	q 8 hours (AM, Mid-after
Cardiotonics		noon and HS)
(except diuretics)		
Eye meds		

clines, except doxycycline or minocycline, completely binds the tetracycline in the gut. Antacids or dairy products are also to be avoided within one hour before or two hours after all tetracyclines are given. Similar precautions are necessary with two newer oral antibiotics, Noroxin® and Cipro®.

In the case of the erythromycins, some may be given closer to food or with antacids without loss of significant amounts of drug absorption. Again, sufficient water must be given to dilute the drug as it disintegrates and dissolves in the GI tract. Most other antibiotics, such as the penicillins and cephalosporins, may be taken without regard to meals. Some antimicrobials, such as sulfas (Gantanol®) or sulfa combinations (Septra®/Bactrim®) and nitrofurantoins (Furadantin®/Macrodantin®) and griseofulvins (Grisactin®), have to be given with food to minimize GI irritation and maximize absorption.

Antacids must be given one to three hours after meals both to be effective and to prevent binding drugs such as tetracyclines, iron, calcium and zinc salts, Noroxin®, Cipro®, Lanoxin®, and other drugs that may be given in small doses (e.g., Sansert®). In addition, it makes no sense to give antacids with meals, as the meal is a far greater buffer to stomach acid than the antacid or Carafate® could be, and maximal stomach secretion of acid occurs 90-120 minutes

Table 13-4

Dosing Interval/Schedule Change or Simplification Cases Noted

Problem	Number	Solution
Antibiotic dosed with meals rather than before meals as ordered	8	Increase po fluids, reschedule to ac if caught in time
Antacids with meals and meds	6	Make antacids pass 1-2 hours after meals/meds
Antipsychotics/Antidepressants dosed 3 to 4 times daily	6	Give single dose at 5-9PM
Antibiotic dosed TID as 9-1-5 rather than over longer period	4	Give morning, midafternoon and bedtime doses

after the start of the meal. This is the reason why H_2 antagonists given during the day should be given at the start of or just before the meal (e.g., Tagamet®, Zantac®, Pepcid®, Axid®). The most rational time to give these drugs, however, is at bedtime, as most stomach ulceration occurs during the night.

Antipsychotics and antidepressants have long periods of pharmacologic effect, and there is no real basis for dosing most antipsychotics (Mellaril®, Serentil®, Thorazine®) on more than a single daily dose. In the case of the sedating or nonsedating antipsychotics (Haldol® and Navane®), the dose should be given around 5 to 7 PM to allow for maximal effect at the "sundowning" period and to allow these agents to induce sleep in 2 to 3 hours. Similar concerns are found for the use of sedating antidepressants (Elavil®/Endep®, Ludiomil®, Sinequan®/Adapin®) given in the morning; the single dose should be moved to the 7 to 9 PM period to allow sedation to ease the patient into sleep. Otherwise, the patient who is sedated early in the day may sleep before the intended bedtime and reverse his sleep cycle, as well as decrease the likelihood of going to sleep in the evening.

The next most common scheduling problem was the administration of antibiotics dosed three times a day on a q 4 h schedule for 9-1-5, rather than before breakfast, midafternoon, and bedtime. Other drugs with short half-lives, such as Pronestyl®, Inderal®, oral nitrates (Isordil®, Sorbitrate®, Peritrate®), scheduled TID should be given on a similar schedule of morning, midafternoon, and bedtime.

A 100% compliance rate was noted with dosing interval or schedule change recommendations made by the consultant pharmacist.

CONCLUSIONS AND IMPLICATIONS

This chapter shows that in one nursing home, problems of inappropriate drug scheduling and administration can commonly occur. If a consultant pharmacist or a provider pharmacist with hospital training schedules the drugs as they should be given, there is still cause for concern when those orders and schedules are not adhered to in the facility. In this study, the consultant, who visited the nursing home monthly, discovered that most problems were due to poor follow-up with the scheduling and intended administration schedule. The PAC survey for medication errors and the federal standards, otherwise known as the indicators for drug monitoring and regimen review, must be followed and monitored by the consultant and provider pharmacists, administrator, director of nursing, and charge nurses to ensure the safest and most efficacious use of medications. While the present study cannot be assumed to be representative of all nursing homes, scheduling and administration of medications is a problem for consideration by nursing home administrators, medical directors, attending physicians, directors of nursing, and pharmacists working in long-term care facilities. Figure 13-1 is a checklist for appropriate drug scheduling.

Figure 13-1
A Checklist for Appropriate Drug Scheduling

1. Are all drugs scheduled before, with or after meals as appropriate ?

2. Are all drugs given with an appropriate interval,e.g. Should TID antibiotics be q 8 h, as 6AM-2PM-10PM, rather than 9-1-5.?

3. Are QID drugs given 9-1-5-9 or should they be q 6 h, e.g. quinidine, antibiotics, Inderal ?

4. Are BID drugs more appropriately q 12 h, especially if they are sustained released drugs such as TheBID, Quinidex Extentabs, Ornade, etc.?

REFERENCES

1. Federal Indicators for Drug Regimen Review. Transmittal No. 174, DHHS, HCFA, State Operators Manual-Provider Certification.

2. Cooper JW. Drug therapy monitoring guidelines. Consultant Press, Watkinsville, GA, 1991.

Chapter 14

The Use of Drugs for No Established Need or Diagnoses in Nursing Home Patients

SUMMARY. The use of drugs without stated diagnoses was studied in a nursing home over a two-year period. There were 21 cases found related to possible presence of dementia (6), extrapyramidal symptoms (4), depression (4), seizures (4), hypokalemia (2), and antithyroid drug propylthiouracil being used for no history of hyperthyroidism (1). The apparent failure to document therapeutic purpose in a problem list or progress notes or to verify need from history, physical, or lab examination were the reasons most commonly noted for these drug-related problems. There is a tendency to prescribe drugs for signs and symptoms in nursing home patients rather than for a documented diagnosis.

INTRODUCTION

The tendency to prescribe drugs for vague and ill-defined problems is a further drug-related problem found in the nursing home. This chapter describes the findings of this problem and gives methods for preventing or detecting and solving this type of DRP.[1]

OPERATIONAL DEFINITIONS

The lack of a verified diagnosis or need for a drug was established if any of the following were noted in a patient's chart:

1. Drugs were ordered "as needed for X symptom or Y sign";

2. Any drug was ordered for a patient without a diagnosis or need stated in a problem list, progress notes, admission, or subsequent history and physical or laboratory test.

RESULTS AND CASE DISCUSSION

Table 14-1 indicates the results found in this study. As noted in Chapter 3, there were only five cases where the drug was stopped by the attending physician when the lack of established diagnosis or demonstrated therapeutic need was found. In other words, the prescriber believed less than one-fourth of the time that the failure to establish need was any reason to stop the medication. In ten cases, the prescriber did add a notation to the progress notes to attempt to justify the need for a medication. Several cases illustrate this DRP.

Antipsychotics

A 78-year-old white female had an order for Mellaril® 25 mg TID "prn agitation." The question was raised by the consultant pharmacist as to whether there was a documented history of dementia, as none could be found in the chart, and a family member had

Table 14-1

No Established Need/Diagnosis

but Drug Therapy Ordered or Ordered Incorrectly

Drug Ordered	Absent Problems, Diagnosis or History	Number (%)	
Antipsychotics	Senile Dementia	6	(28.6)
Anticholinergics	Extrapyramidal	4	(19.1)
Antidepressant	Ordered "PRN Depression"	4	(19.1)
Anticonvulsant	No Seizure	4	(19.1)
Potassium Supplement	No Diuretic or history of hypokalemia	2	(9.5)
Propylthiouracil	No hyperthyroidism	1	(4.8)
		21	(100.0)

stated that the patient seemed to be more disoriented since entering the facility and receiving almost daily doses of Mellaril®. The physician refused to stop the Mellaril® and increased the dose to TID regular schedule until the patient was continually sedated, developed three decubitus ulcers, and died from decubitus-related sepsis within six weeks after the Mellaril® was started.

Anticholinergics

Many prescribers irrationally begin a patient on an anticholinergic when drugs such as Haldol®, which have the possibility of causing extrapyramidal symptoms (EPS), are started. The preferred method of using anticholinergics is not to begin these drugs until definite EPS are noted. An 83-year-old black male was started on Haldol® 1 mg BID and Cogentin® 1 mg BID at the same time, with resultant anticholinergic toxicity of dry mouth, urinary retention, and obstipation. When the consultant pharmacist questioned the prescriber's use of the Cogentin®, the Cogentin® was stopped, with improvement in all symptoms of anticholinergic toxicity.

Antidepressants

Antidepressants have to be continuously used for three to four weeks at therapeutic doses in order to be effective for documented or suspected depression. The use of antidepressants "as needed for depression," does not give the drugs a chance to help the patients if needed. A 69-year-old recently bereaved widow appeared to have difficulty sleeping several weeks after her husband's funeral. Doxepin® 75 mg "prn depression" was ordered for bedtime use. On pharmacist questioning of the order and observation that the patient was sleeping one to two hours after all three meals, a change in post-prandial sleep to activity was tried with success after the Doxepin® was stopped.

Anticonvulsants

Chronic seizures are not a common problem in nursing home patients. Some patients who have had a stroke may have had an isolated seizure at the time of the stoke, but these seizures are usually not chronic in nature. The same effect may be noted for the patient with a history of alcohol abuse (i.e., the patient may have had a single episode of seizure when drying out). Patients on anticonvulsants with no verifiable history of seizures may need a cautious trial of gradual withdrawal of the seizure medication, especially if they have a subtherapeutic serum level of the drug. A 78-year-old white male with no history of stroke, seizure, or alcoholism was noted to be on Dilantin® 100 mg 3 times a day with a subtherapeutic level of 2.7 mcg/ml. When the prescriber was made aware of the situation, he ordered the Dilantin® decreased to 100 mg twice a day for one week, then decreased further to 100 mg at bedtime for the next week with observation for seizure activity on each shift. No problems were noted with this withdrawal schedule.

Potassium Supplements

Many times potassium supplements are ordered continued when a diuretic is stopped, or they are simply not discontinued when the diuretic is stopped. It is not rational to have a patient on a potassium supplement when no diuretic is being used. In both cases, however, when the patient's potassium levels were checked, the levels were not outside normal, so the prescriber declined to stop a drug that is the most lethal drug used in the hospital setting when used by the intravenous route. In one case, this was nearly fatal. An 87-year-old black female who became dehydrated with furosemide had this drug stopped, but her KCl was continued. On questioning, the prescriber ordered a serum potassium, which came back at 4.7 mEq/L one week after the furosemide was stopped. Two months later, the consultant pharmacist was asked to look at the patient, who had become progressively stuporous with pulses 36-48 BPM. A stat serum potassium was 7.5 mEq/L. Any level over 5-6 mEq/L is considered toxic. The KCl was stopped and Kayexalate® was started for one week to lower her total body potassium. One week later it was 4.3 mEq/L, and her pulse had risen to 64-72 BPM. The patient's orientation to time, place, and person had markedly improved at this time.

Antithyroid Drug

A patient with no history of hyperthyroidism was found on propylthiouracil, with no signs or symptoms of hypo- or hyper-thyroidism. Despite the recommendation that lab work to confirm need for the drug be done, the attending physician refused on the basis that his palpation of the patient's neck had detected a goiter (which could be present in either too low or too high thyroid levels). Thyroid disease is never confirmed without a thyroid profile of lab tests.

IMPLICATIONS

It appears that the use of some drugs lacks therapeutic justification, especially where the physician has failed to document a diagnosis or finding. Both health care practitioners and patients and their families need to be aware of the need to question the use of drugs in the nursing home patient and to challenge improper use when it is suspected, as in Figure 14-1.

Figure 14-1
A Checklist for The Appropriate Establishment of Diagnoses

1. Are there orders for symptoms or signs, rather than specific diagnoses ?

2. Are there duplicative orders for the same symptoms, e.g. "...agitation, ...apprehension, ...anxiety, ... restlessness.." that may pertain to the same problem ?

3. Are as needed orders not used in a month to 60 days; if so they should be discontuinued.

4. Does the attending physician address the need for each order,or does the nurse initiate many new order changes ?

5. Does the consultant pharmacist attempt to recommend elimination of drugs symptomatically ordered or duplicated.?

REFERENCE

1. Cooper JW. Drug-related problems in a geriatric long term care facility. *J Ger Drug Ther* 1986; 1(1):47-68.

Chapter 15

Patient Refusal and Inability to Take Medications in a Nursing Home

SUMMARY. Nursing home patients have the right to refuse to take their medications. They also may encounter difficulty in the administration of their medications that may or may not be overcome by patient counseling. Eighteen cases of patient refusal or inability to take medications were noted in a nursing home over a two-year period. Patient-perceived problems in taking medications, patient belief that the medication was not needed, or conscious fear of taking the medication were the most common reasons for refusal. Facilities, as well as patients and their families and health care practitioners, need to understand both their rights and the ramifications of refusal to take medications. The prescriber attempted to address the problem of patient refusal by changing drug dosage form or discontinuing the refused medication in 5 of 18 cases.

INTRODUCTION

Failure to take medications as prescribed is a drug-related problem with many implications.[1] Patients may experience real difficulty in attempting to take oral medications (e.g., cannot swallow). Alternative dosage forms, such as the use of liquid rather than solid capsules or tablets, may help overcome this difficulty in swallowing. Patients may consciously believe that they are having an adverse reaction to medication, whether this is the case or a psychosomatic reaction to their illness, the need for treatment, and/or their environment. For example, ambulatory patients taking NSAI drugs for their arthritis may experience gastric discomfort and stop taking the medication before serious gastric erosion, anemia, or acute gastrointestinal bleeding occurs. The nursing home patient may not be as likely to pinpoint the reason why he does not want to take the medication, due to decreased mentation.

Perhaps the most important reason patients may deliberately fail to take a drug, however, is that they do not perceive the need for, or agree to the use of, one or more of their medications. Patient and family or responsible party counseling on the need for medication compliance, as well as the careful consideration of therapeutic alternatives, is vital in ensuring that the most efficacious and least toxic drug therapy needed is, in fact, used in the patient.

The purpose of this chapter is to present patient refusal to take drugs in the context of patient rights and facility and health care practitioner responsibilities.

PATIENT REFUSAL DETECTION METHODS

The refusal of patients to take their drugs was noted by a consultant pharmacist from the nursing home medication administration record (MAR), nurse's notes in the patient's chart, the nurse bringing the refusal to the consultant pharmacist's attention, and/or the pharmacy dispensing records for individual patients. Whenever a failure to take medication as prescribed was noted, the consultant pharmacist attempted to recommend a change in dosage form or drug to encourage compliant patient behavior. A notation of prescriber response to recommendation and patient acceptance of change when authorized was made.

RESULTS AND CASE DISCUSSION

The results of this drug-related problem investigation are noted in Table 15-1. In only 5 of the 18 cases was an attempt made by the attending physician to change drug therapy after the consultant pharmacist made a recommendation. In all other cases except for insulin, the patient refusal eventually led to the discontinuance of

Table 15-1

Patient Refusal/Inability to Take Medication

Type	Problem (Complaint)	Number	(%)
Bulk Laxative	Refusal ("Can't Swallow")	5	(27.8)
Hypnotic	Refusal ("Don't need")	4	(22.2)
Stimulant	Refusal ("Makes me excited")	3	(16.7)
Multiple Vitamin	Unable to swallow ("gags;nauseates")	3	(16.7)
Insulin	Refusal	1	(5.6)
Quinidine	Refusal	1	(5.6)
Sublingual NTG	Refusal	1	(5.6)
	total	18	(100.0)

the drug, without physician accordance. Illustrative composite cases give resolution recommendations and results.

Bulk Laxative Refusal

Most patients who refused bulk laxatives of psyllium (e.g., Metamucil®) had real difficulty in swallowing the suspended particles of the laxative and were not used to drinking the volume of fluid necessary to ensure the safe use of bulk laxatives. All patients were incontinent of their urine and consciously restricted their fluid intake, which made the use of bulk laxatives unsafe. A recommendation of milk of magnesia was accepted in three of the five cases by physician and patient.

Sleeping Medication Refusal

In all cases, the patients' refusal was based on their perception that they "did not need any sleeping pill." In fact, all cases were errors in recopying orders for sleep medications that had been routinely started on an as needed (prn) basis.

Stimulant Drug Refusal

Again, in all cases, the patients or their families wanted to know why the patients needed the stimulant Ritalin®. The physician response was that the drug was being used as an antidepressant or to counter the effects of nightly long-acting sleeping medication (e.g., Dalmane®). None of the drugs was stopped despite consistent patient refusal to take the drug.

Vitamin Refusal

In two of the three cases, the tablet was given on an empty stomach. A change to giving the vitamin tablet with the largest meal of the day overcame refusal. In the third case, a liquid vitamin had to be used due to swallowing difficulty with the therapeutic vitamin tablet.

Needed Drug Refusal

In the case of the insulin-dependent diabetic patient refusing insulin, a choice was given to the patient: either accept the medication injections or leave the facility. This approach produced acceptance of the insulin injections. In the case of quinidine, refusal due to persistent nausea and diarrhea led to discontinuance of the quinidine, with subsequent patient improvement. The substitute of a nitroglycerin patch for the sublingual led to acceptance of the needed medication.

DISCUSSION

Patients have the right to know about their disease states, their drugs, and their prognosis, with or without treatment. Physicians have a right to expect compliant patient behavior with their therapeutic orders. Nurses administer and observe therapeutic order effects, and pharmacist consultants should encourage compliant drug-taking or find alternatives in drug or dosage form to ensure optimal drug therapeutic outcome. Nursing home administrators attempt to ensure that the patients and their families or responsible parties are compliant with therapeutic orders and to resolve refusal situations so that all persons are protected. Any patient refusal to take a medication should be pursued to a satisfactory resolution, even if the patient has the right to refuse life-saving drugs or nutrition.

The "living will" concept of no unusual means to prolong life was not studied, nor were "no code" order patients included in this study. The only checklist for this chapter is to see that the patient's rights and the inherent responsibilities of the prescribers, facility, nurses, and pharmacists are followed.

REFERENCE

1. Cooper JW. Drug-related problems in a geriatric long term care facility. *J Ger Drug Ther* 1986; 1(1):46-68.

Chapter 16

Drug Changes Needed in Nursing Home Patients

SUMMARY. Drug changes needed to improve the quality of nursing home pharmacotherapy were studied in a nursing home over a two-year period as part of a larger study of drug-related problems. Nine cases of consultant pharmacist-recommended changes in drug therapy were noted, with prescriber change made in four of the nine cases. The most common needed changes involved the continuous use of long-acting benzodiazepines (3), nitroglycerin ointment used as needed for chest pain (2), cimetidine full dose therapy for longer than six to eight weeks (2), continuous full dose trimethoprim/sulfamethoxazole (1), and potassium gluconate in a case of potassium chloride deficiency.

INTRODUCTION AND METHODS

The use of less than optimal drug therapy in nursing home patients has many facets. Less than optimal drug therapy could be:

1. The wrong drug for a given diagnosis;
2. The wrong drug for a given patient condition or contraindication;
3. The wrong dosage form to achieve a therapeutic goal;
4. The wrong length of therapy or stop order period;
5. The wrong dose of a given drug;
6. The wrong length of therapy with a given dosage schedule; or
7. Any concurrent combination of 1-6.

This study considered monthly the drug therapy of nursing home patients via a process outlined in Chapter 2.[1]

RESULTS AND COMPOSITE CASE DISCUSSION

Table 16-1 indicates the results found over a two-year period of intensive monthly drug regimen review by a consultant pharmacist. Composite case discussions by therapeutic class give a better understanding of this type of drug-related problem.

Continuous Long-Acting Benzodiazepines

The continuous use of the longer-acting sedatives/hypnotics Valium®, Librium®, Dalmane®, Tranxene®, Azene®, Paxipam®, and Centrax® is associated with the development of pseudodementia,

Table 16-1

Dosing Modification, Length of Therapy

or Drug Change Needed

Problem	Recommendation	Number	(%)
Continuous long acting Benzodiazepines	Oxazepam or Lorazepam	3	(33.3)
Nitroglycen (NTG) Ointment "PRN Chest Pain	Sublinqual NTG	2	(22.2)
Cimetidine Full Dose Therapy longer than 8 weeks	400 mg qIIS	1	(11.1)
Trimethoprim/Sulfamthoxazole double strength twice a day continuous schedule	Decrease dose to one-half tablet HS in CUTI	1	(11.1)
K-Gluconate in hypokalemic, hypochloremic metabolic alkalosis due to thiazide diuretic	KCl	1	(11.1)
	total	9	(100.0)

depression, and an increased frequency of falls. In all cases, the use of a shorter-acting sedative or hypnotic (e.g., Serax®, Ativan®, Xanax®, Halcion®, or Restoril®) was recommended, with limited physician and patient acceptance. The use of any sedative for longer than 3-4 months or any sleeping medication for longer than 7-14 days on a continuous basis is not recommended by standard references. Unfortunately, patient dependence and family desire that the patient not be withdrawn led to no changes in this category.

Nitroglycerin Ointment "PRN Chest Pain"

In both cases, the prescriber was informed that the ointment takes 30-60 minutes to give effective relief of chest pain. A continuous administration schedule of ointment, patch, or sublingual dosage form was made, with no changes evident. One of the patients continued to experience daily chest pain after meals and died of natural causes, which included chest pain at the time of death. The other patient's family changed physicians after discussion with the charge nurse and consultant pharmacist of the physician's reluctance to order rational drug therapy.

Continuous Full-Dose Cimetidine Therapy

The manufacturer recommends and many clinical studies verify that full-dose therapy in confirmed peptic ulcer disease is not necessary for longer than six to eight weeks. In neither case was a change made, with a resultant cost of drug four times greater than needed.

Continuous Full-Dose Urinary Anti-infective

Once an acute urinary tract infection is eliminated, a single bedtime dose of trimethoprim alone (50-100 mg) is as effective as either a full dose of the trimethoprim/sulfamethoxazole or bedtime half dose, with much less chance of adverse reaction. This recommendation was ignored by the prescriber.

Wrong Potassium Salt

Most patients who develop low potassium also get low chloride and therefore need potassium chloride rather than potassium gluconate replacement therapy. The one case where the latter drug was used and serum chlorides remained low, the prescriber changed to the chloride, with subsequent improvement in serum chloride.

IMPLICATIONS

This chapter presented some needed changes in drug, dose, dosage form, and schedule. All persons concerned with rational drug therapy should strive for the best possible pharmacotherapy. A checklist for rational assessment is found in Figure 16-1.

Figure 16-1

A Checklist for Drug Usage Quality Assessment

1. Is each drug given in the lowest possible effective dose.?

2. Is each drug given for the appropriate length of time ?

3. Is the best drug from the theapeutic class, e.g. shortest-

acting for most drugs, being prescribed?

4. Is the correct dosage form being utilized ?

5. Is each drugs effect being assessed by the nurse, physi-

cian and pharmacist?

REFERENCE

1. Cooper JW. Drug-related problems in a geriatric long term care facility. *J Ger Drug Ther* 1986; 1(1):47-68.

Chapter 17

Drug-Related Problems in the Elderly Nursing Home Patient: Present Knowledge, Future Research Needs

SUMMARY. This book has dealt with the specific drug-related problems of elderly nursing home patients within the nursing home environment. This chapter summarizes the findings of this text and poses questions yet to be resolved. There should be significant funding initiatives to find cost-effective methods to prevent and decrease the frequency of DRPs. The determination of methods and demonstration of method efficacy should be among the highest priority goals of gerontology and geriatrics education and research programs.

INTRODUCTION

Pharmacotherapy is the most frequently used and supposedly most cost-effective treatment modality in the elderly. Drug-related problems (DRPs) may be defined as any unwanted consequence of the drug use process. Although many events can and do occur in this process, from the assessment of a patient's problems to the therapeutic outcome in that patient, the two main DRP classifications are drug misuse and adverse drug reaction or interaction. When both types of problems are simultaneously assessed in the same patient population entering a hospital, the frequency of those problems has been demonstrated to increase with age.[1]

Geriatric pharmacy practice in the United States of America was mandated with the development of the nursing home industry after the 1965 passage of Title XVIII and XIX of the Social Security

Administration Act. The Medicaid and Medicare provisions of this act allowed the private sector to foster a generally for-profit industry, with its positive and negative aspects. The exposure of these abuses led, in great measure, to the regulatory inclusion and expansion of the pharmacist's role in the care of the geriatric patient, also known as consultant pharmacy. The February 1974 *Federal Register* states that the pharmacist should "monitor the drug regimen . . . monthly" in all nursing home patients. This expansion led directly to an increased level of pharmacy services in both drug distribution and clinical service areas. The need for and effects of pharmacist-conducted drug regimen reviews in long-term care facilities have been studied by several investigators.[1-16] A paper in 1987 summarized the financial impact of pharmacist drug regimen reviews on drug use from 15 previously published studies.[17] Comprehensive studies of drug distribution in nursing homes have repeatedly demonstrated the safety and cost-savings of modified unit-dose systems.[14,18,19]

DRP-REDUCTION BY THE CONSULTANT PHARMACIST IN LONG-TERM CARE

Admissions to Nursing Homes

The cost-savings resulting from the involvement of consultant pharmacists in health care of patients in geriatric long-term care facilities has found that over half of patients admitted to a long-term care facility were found to have drug-related problems that influenced their need for admission to the nursing home. On average, three drug-related problems were detected per patient. Drug class duplication, unnecessary drug therapy, newly identified problems, suspected adverse drug reactions, and laboratory data needed to assess therapy were the most significant problems.[20]

Cost-Reduction Potential. If one-half of nursing home admissions could be prevented or delayed by consultant pharmacist intervention in the ambulatory setting, what would be the cost-savings to the health care system?

Medication Errors

This book documents that once patients are admitted to a nursing home, almost two-thirds of rigorous drug regimen reviews detect significant drug-related problems (DRPs) over a two-year period. Three-fourths of the DRP solution recommendations were implemented by the attending physician. Medication errors related to a poor distribution system were the most common problem. Modified unit-dose systems have been shown to reduce these errors, but many state reimbursement systems do not allow for unit-dose system reimbursement. Yet these systems pay for hospital admissions caused by the omission of the needed medication.[14,18,19]

Cost-Reduction Potential. If unit-dose systems were to become the standard of care for long-term care as they have become for the acute-care hospital, more medication errors could be detected earlier, and it is likely that fewer serious medication errors would occur. (Please see Chapter 4 for more discussion.)

Adverse Drug Reactions

The next most common DRP in this book was adverse drug reactions and interactions and relative contraindications to drug use that led to adverse drug reactions. Almost two-thirds of these adverse drug reactions were preventable in that careful attention to the patient's complete history and problem list should have resulted in drug changes/discontinuances. By accepting the consultant pharmacist's recommendations, this nursing home saved the health care system over $163,000 in adverse drug reaction treatment costs over a 2-year period.[21]

Cost Reduction Potential. If up to two-thirds of adverse drug reactions in nursing home patients could be prevented by intensive drug regimen review and patient assessment, could adverse drug reaction-related hospitalizations for problems such as digoxin toxicity, NSAID-associated gastrointestinal bleeding, and psychotropic drug-associated falls and fractures be reduced? (Please see Chapters 5 and 6 for specific problems.)

Interruption of Clinical Services

A five-year study has shown that when a consultant pharmacist is retained, fired, and then rehired, drugs per patient, admission, death, and hospitalization rates change in a predictable fashion.[22] When the consultant was hired, drug costs were cut in half, with similar reductions in drug-related problems, hospitalizations, and overall mortality over a two-year period. When the consultant was fired, drug costs doubled, DRPs and death rates increased over one year. When the consultant was rehired (only because of a state regulatory threat to close the facility because of poor drug use control), drug costs and related problems were reduced over a two-year period. An 11:1 cost justification ratio was observed for drug cost reduction alone, divided by consultant reimbursement between periods.

Cost Reduction Potential. Reduced hospitalizations, reduced drug costs, and reduced adverse reactions, as well as increased rehabilitation, are potential areas for cost reduction.

Drug Therapy Management Considerations

Can a clinical consultant pharmacist manage the total drug therapy of nursing home patients? Compared to a control group that received traditional patient care, the prescribing pharmacist's group had a significantly lower number of deaths, drugs, and hospitalizations. With physician supervision and consent, it appears that the practice of having consultant clinical pharmacists prescribe drug therapy and render general care has the potential for saving the health care system approximately $70,000 per year per 100 skilled nursing facility beds.[23] The number of drugs per patient can be shown to be decreased by a consultant pharmacist's services. The pharmacist can also qualitatively improve the detection, diagnosis, and resultant pharmacotherapy of nursing home patients. With acceptance of a consultant pharmacist's recommendations, improved control of high blood pressure, congestive heart failure and atrial fibrillation, arthritis and related pain, anemia and malnutrition, psychiatric problems, seizures, constipation, and eye and urinary tract infections, has been demonstrated.[24-34] An additional cost-savings concept was made apparent in the last study.[34] Health care costs can be greatly reduced by using a lower level of care. Specifically, a cost savings of over $1,200 per injectable aminoglycoside treatment episode for urinary tract infections was shown when patients were dosed and followed in a nursing home rather than in the hospital setting that was used before this study was conducted. (Please see Chapters 7-12.)

Cost Reduction Potential. Decreased medication, lab tests, and (potentially) physician fees, can result if a pharmacist can better manage long-term care patients than the current system of care for these patients. A lower level of care option is another way to save costs.

ALTERNATIVES TO NURSING HOME CARE

Patients can be treated at lower levels of care with substantial cost savings, as there are several less expensive alternatives to nursing home care. Home health care is a debatably cost-effective alternative to either acute or long-term care. Several studies have found a significant number of drug-related problems in this population, yet over 90% of home health care agencies appear to receive pharmacy services.[35-37]

In a study of day-care elderly patients, over half of this population had significant DRPs that were not detected by their prescribers or the day-care workers who were administering their drugs, and all patients were on waiting lists for admission to skilled or intermediate care facilities.[38] The patients were in a holding pattern, waiting for a long-term care bed, and had medication-associated problems that could have been detected and resolved with better preventive care. On examination of the apparent effects of diagnosis-related group (DRG) reimbursement patterns in acute care facilities, the anecdotal opinion of many long-term care facility professionals is that many patients are being prematurely "dumped" in nursing homes. This may occur in some instances when a patient's Medicare hospital days, personal, or other third-party coverage is exhausted.

Swing beds are another alternative for either hospital or nursing home bed use or as a step before nursing home care. They have also been tried as an alternative to nursing home placement. Our recent experience is that these are generally extremely sick or terminal patients who have used all their Medicare hospital days, have high overall treatment costs, and have a great number of drug-related problems (DRPs).[39] Curiously, the swing bed reimbursement rate was almost one-third lower than the per diem for the adjacent skilled nursing facility, with no additional drug coverage for the swing bed patient, yet drug costs alone per patient were almost three times greater for swing bed than skilled nursing facility patients in the first week of an average three-week length of stay for the swing bed patients. All swing bed patients had an average of 1.7 DRPs during their 20-day stay, which was almost 3 times the DRP prevalence rate found on monthly drug regimen review in a concurrent study conducted in the adjacent nursing home.[21]

Therapeutic Substitution

Therapeutic substitution may produce cost savings in the care of the geriatric long-term care patient. In terms of savings to third-party programs, several findings are notable. The therapeutic substitution of acetaminophen or enteric-coated aspirin on a regular dosage schedule in place of more expensive NSAIDs has been shown to save $330-$350 per patient per year in drug costs alone.[40] The costs of treating the anemia and gastrointestinal bleeding associated with NSAIDs and ASA (the more expensive therapy) may be more than money: they may extend to mortality, which is difficult to measure in terms of value.[27] The use of skim milk and milk shakes in place of the more expensive enteral feeding supplements has been shown to save almost $1,000 per patient per year.[40]

Cost Reduction Potential. If the consultant pharmacist's therapeutic substitution recommendations are accepted, further cost savings may be realized in overall health care costs.

REDUCTION OF DRUG MONITORING COSTS

A recent study found that when the consultant pharmacist ordered selected lab tests in preference to routine lab tests, a cost savings of almost $500 per patient per year in lab test costs was realized. Over 90% of the consultant-ordered lab tests produced significant results, while less than 5% of the routine tests produced clinically useful information.[41] By recommending the discontinuance of routine urine sugar and acetone (S&As) tests, which produce little useful information, the consultant pharmacist has been shown to save $337 per diabetic patient per year in the nursing home setting.[42] On the other hand, it has been recommended that if a geriatric long-term care patient is to receive NSAIDs or ASA therapy, the hemoglobin and hematocrit should be monitored on a more frequent, perhaps every two-months, basis.[27]

Cost Reduction Potential. If the cost of any health care expenditure can be justified as clinically relevant and preventing serious adverse effects of drugs, the overall cost must be considered.

FUTURE DRUG-RELATED PROBLEMS RESEARCH AREAS

There remain a number of questions to be resolved abut DRPs and consultant pharmacist practice in nursing homes:

1. Should federal and private insurers expand coverage of nursing home and ambulatory care of geriatric patients to include clinical services as well as intravenous therapy and additives and nutritional therapy?
2. Should private nursing home patients receive a different quality of care than public-supported patients?[43]
3. Should consultant pharmacists receive a separate payment for their services, just as the physician, rather than negotiate their fee with nursing home administrators out of the patient per diem? There is anecdotal evidence that there is an economic disadvantage to the consultant to decrease drugs per patient and drug-related problems when he receives minimal to no reimbursement for consultant services and also loses prescription revenue. A less preferable alternative to consider is whether the consultant and vendor services should be separated by professional, regulatory, and/or ethical bases.
4. Should consultant pharmacists have greater responsibility for the total therapeutic management of nursing home patients, to include prescribing and ordering of lab tests?

5. Should boards of pharmacy move to require a rigorous educational process and certification for consultant pharmacists in their respective states?
6. Should the Doctor of Pharmacy be the entry-level degree for the practice of pharmacy, and should geriatric patient training be a mandated educational experience?

SUMMARY RECOMMENDATIONS

In summary, the recommendations for reduction of drug-related problems in nursing home patients include provision of:

1. A tightly-controlled drug distribution system that accounts for all doses and treatments given to patients and state or other third-party reimbursement for these cost-effective and safer drug distribution systems;
2. Rigorous drug regimen review that detects and reduces drug-related problems and qualitatively improves pharmacotherapy by all health care practitioners;
3. Expanded and different reimbursement support mechanisms for patients' medications and consultant services;
4. Further studies to conclusively demonstrate the cost savings of consultant pharmacy practice;
5. Expanded educational requirements for those pharmacists who desire to provide consultant services; and
6. A more comprehensive set of drug regimen review standards and guidelines than the current minimal indicators.

A review of consulting with long-term care patients has been published previously.[44] A more stringent drug regimen review guidelines and home study certification course has been established.[45]

REFERENCES

1. Eckel FM, Latiolais CJ. An analysis of pharmaceutical service in forty-one nursing homes. *Am J Hosp Pharm* 1964; 21:351-360.
2. McLeod DC, Eckel FM. Relationship between method of reimbursement

and scope of pharmacy service in nursing homes. *J Am Pharm Assoc* 1969; NS9:62-64.

3. Eckel FM, Crawley HK. A study of pharmacy services in North Carolina rest homes. *J Am Pharm Assoc* 1971; NS11:387-390.

4. Eckel FM. Improving system didn't help—but change to unit dose did. *Modern Nursing Home* 1971; 71(Sept.):10-16.

5. Crawley HK, Eckel FM, McLeod DC. Comparison of a traditional and unit-dose system in a nursing home. *Drug Intell Clin Pharm* 1971; 5:166-171.

6. Townsend C. Old Age—the last segregation. Grossman Publishers, New York, 1971.

7. Anon. Nursing home care in the United States; Failure in public policy. Supporting papers series. U.S. Congress Special Committee on Aging, United States Senate, Sub-Committee on Long Term Care, 1974-1978.

8. Anon. Long term care facility improvement study. Introductory report. DHEW Pub. No.(05) 76-50021, 1975.

9. Anon. Physician's prescribing patterns in skilled nursing facilities. LTCF improvement campaign monograph No.2 DHEW Pub. No.(05) 76-50050, 1976.

10. Anon. Problems remain in reviews of Medicaid-financed drug therapy in nursing homes. Report to the Congress by the Comptroller General. Pub. No. HRD-80-56, 1980.

11. Cheung A, Kayne R. An application of clinical pharmacy in extended care facilities. *Calif Pharm* 1975; 23:22-25.

12. Thompson J, Floyd R. Cost-analysis of comprehensive consultant pharmacist services in the skilled nursing facility: a progress report. *Calif Pharm* 1978; 26:22-26.

13. Cooper JW, Bagwell CG. Contribution of the consultant pharmacist to national drug usage in the long-term care facility. *J Am Ger Soc* 1978; 26:513-520.

14. Strandberg LR, Dawson GW, Mathieson D et al. Effect of comprehensive pharmaceutical services on drug use in long-term care facilities. *Am J Hosp Pharm* 1980; 37:92-94.

15. Witte KW, Leeds NH, Pathak DS et al. Drug-regimen review in skilled nursing facilities by consulting clinical pharmacists. *Am J Hosp Pharm* 1980; 37:820-824.

16. McGhan WF, Wertheimer AI, Martilla JK. Assessing the need for pharmacist-conducted drug regimen reviews in skilled nursing and intermediate care facilities. *Contemp Pharm Pract* 1980; 3:203-209.

17. McGhan WF, Einarson TR, Sabers DL et al. A meta-analysis of the impact of pharmacist drug regimen reviews in long-term care facilities. *J Ger Drug Ther* 1987; 1(3):23-35.

18. Barker KN, Mikeal RL, Pearson RE. Medication errors in nursing homes and small hospitals. *Am J Hosp Pharm* 1982; 39:987-991.

19. Strandberg L, Stennett D. Drug distribution systems in Oregon's long term care facilities. *Hosp Form* 1981; 29:627-637.

20. Cooper JW. Effects of intensive consultant pharmacy review of nursing home admission orders. *Consult Pharm* 1987; 2:152-155.

21. Cooper JW. Drug-related problems in a geriatric long term care facility. *J Ger Drug Ther* 1986; 1(1):47-68.

22. Cooper JW. Effect of initiation, termination and reinitiation of consultant clinical pharmacists services in a geriatric long term care facility. *Med Care* 1985; 23:84-88.

23. Thompson JF, McGhan WF, Ruffalo RL et al. Clinical pharmacists prescribing drug therapy in a geriatric setting: outcome of a trial. *J Am Ger Soc* 1984; 32:154-159.

24. Williamson DH, Cooper JW, Kotzan JA. Consultant pharmacist impact on hypertension therapy in a geriatric long term care facility. *Hosp Form* 1984; 19:123-128.

25. Pink LA, Cooper JW, Francis WR. Digoxin-related communications in a long term care facility. *Nursing Homes* 1985; 34:25-31.

26. Wilcher DE, Cooper JW. Consultant pharmacist effect on analgesic/anti-inflammatory usage in a geriatric long term care facility. *J Am Ger Soc* 1981; 29:429-432.

27. Cooper JW, Mallet L, Wade WE. Anemia prevalence and treatment outcomes in a geriatric long term care facilities population. *J Pharmacoepid* 1990; 1(1):61-70.

28. Cooper JW, Cobb HH. Nutritional correlates and outcomes in a geriatric long term care facility. *Nutr Supp Serv* 1988; 8(8):5-7.

29. Tsai AE, Cooper JW, McCall CY. Consultant pharmacist effect on hematopoietic and vitamin therapy in a geriatric long term care facility. *Hosp Form* 1982; 17:225-235.

30. Cooper JW, Francisco GE. Psychotropic usage in long term care facility geriatric patients. *Hosp Form* 1981; 16:407-419.

31. Wade WE, Cobb HH. Consultant pharmacist effects on seizure control in an institution for mentally retarded. *Consult Pharm* 1987; 2:156-158.

32. Cooper JW. Chronic constipation correlates and prevention in a geriatric nursing home population. *J Pharmacoepidemiology* 1991; 1(2).

33. Cooper JW. Consultant pharmacist contribution to reduction of eye infections in a geriatric nursing home. *Consult Pharm* 1988; 3:83.

34. Lawler RS, Cooper JW, Kotzan JA. Consultant pharmacist input to treatment of urinary tract infections in a geriatric long term care facility. *Hosp Pharm* 1980; 15:562-572.

35. Cooper JW, Griffin DH, Francisco GE et al. Pharmacist in home health care. *Hosp Form* 1985; 20:643-650.

36. Solomon DK, Baumgartner RP, Weissman AM et al. Pharmaceutical services to improve drug therapy for home health care patients. *Am J Hosp Pharm* 1978; 35:553-557.

37. Szeinbach SL, Bonk DS, Mason HL. Pharmacy involvement in home health care agencies: a national survey. *Consult Pharm* 1987; 2:292-296.

38. Cooper JW. Drug-related problems in geriatric day-care patients. *Consult Pharm* 1988; 3:193.

39. Cooper JW. Swing bed patients and the consultant pharmacist. *Consult Pharm* 1988; 3:287.

40. Cooper JW. Nursing home drug and nutritional therapy cost-savings by the consultant pharmacist. *Nursing Homes* 1987; 36(6):6-8.

41. Cooper JW. Appropriate utilization of laboratory tests in the geriatric nursing home. *Nursing Homes* 1988; 37(4):5-8.

42. Cooper JW. Cost-savings from discontinuance of urinary sugar and acetone tests. *Consult Pharm* 1988; 3:83.

43. Wade WE, Talley SE. Consultant pharmacist effect on private vs. public patients in geriatric nursing homes. *Consult Pharm* 1987; 2:399-403.

44. Cooper JW. Consulting to long term care patients. In: Brown TR, Smith MC, eds. Institutional pharmacy practice. 2nd. ed. Baltimore, Williams and Wilkins 1986, pp. 649-662.

45. Cooper JW. Community and nursing home practice drug therapy and patient education guidelines. Consultant Press, Watkinsville, GA, 1991.

Index